NEW LEFT REVIEW 115

SECOND SERIES

JANUARY FEBRUARY 2019

PROGRAMME NOTES

SUSAN WATKINS: America vs China

Introducing a triptych of perspectives on the PRC, as the drumbeat from Washington grows louder. Is the American imperium now so vast, so overweening in its demands, that any rising power must grate against it?

PETER NOLAN: The CPC and the Ancien Régime

Roots of the PRC's legitimating ideology in the *longue durée* of Chinese history, as source of the Party's confidence that it need not imitate Western models in the coming century. Peter Nolan sets out the view from Zhongnanhai on the desirable relation between market and state—a potential alternative to the current world order?

CHRISTOPHER CONNERY: Ronald Coase in Beijing

On the eve of the financial crisis, Giovanni Arrighi's *Adam Smith in Beijing* posited the advent of a world-equalizing market state in China. Christopher Connery now takes a sardonic look at the country's 'institutional economics' through the eyes of an idiosyncratic English Hayekian.

VICTOR SHIH: China's Credit Conundrum

Interviewed by Robert Brenner, Victor Shih discusses the one-off factors that enabled China's rise as workshop of the world and its subsequent dependence on state credit as driver of growth. Contradictions between the conditions for political and financial stability, as the Xi regime superintends an unsteady slowdown.

FASSIN & DEFOSSEZ: An Improbable Movement?

The policies and pretensions of a Bourbonnais president as background to the political insurgency of provincial France. Origins and complexion of the *gilets jaunes* mobilization, with the Elysée resorting to the worst police violence since May 68.

BURTON & SOMERVILLE: Degrowth: A Defence

Counterblast to Robert Pollin's programme in NLR 112 for a green-growth new deal, arguing that a radical reduction in greenhouse-gas emissions requires a smaller global economy. Proposals for a drastic overhaul of production, construction, transportation and agricultural practices.

LOLA SEATON: Green Questions

A survey of the 'green strategy' debate in recent numbers of NLR unravels the threads of twin disagreements about GDP growth, which appears, by turns, a political-economic necessity and an ecological death-sentence. Steady-state, half-earthing, degrowth, green new deal? All have questions to answer.

BOOK REVIEWS

FREDERIK VAN DAM on Francis Mulhern, *Figures of Catastrophe*. Elegant elucidation of an unsuspected literary genre centred on culture as a ground for social conflict.

ALEXANDRA REZA on Stephen Smith, *La ruée vers Europe*. Projected convergence of African demographic growth and economic stagnation as conditions for a migratory 'scramble for Europe'.

REBECCA LOSSIN on Mauvaise Troupe, *The ZAD and NoTAV*. Oral history and barefoot ethnography combine in a participants' account of territorial struggles in Piedmont and Brittany.

CONTRIBUTORS

MARK BURTON: *scholar-activist at Steady State Manchester;* author of In Place of Growth *(2012)*

CHRISTOPHER CONNERY: *at* UC *Santa Cruz; author of* Empire of the Text *(1998) and co-editor of* The Worlding Project *(2007)*

ANNE-CLAIRE DEFOSSEZ: *researching women in French politics at the Institute for Advanced Study, Princeton*

DIDIER FASSIN: *recent works include* Humanitarian Reason *(2011),* At the Heart of the State *(2015) and* Life: A Critical User's Manual *(2018); at the* IAS, *Princeton*

REBECCA LOSSIN: *doctoral candidate at Columbia University; see also* NLR *107*

PETER NOLAN: *at Cambridge; recent works include* Is China Buying the World? *(2012) and* Understanding China *(2016); see also* NLR *64, 80*

ALEXANDRA REZA: *teaches modern languages at Trinity College, Oxford; see also* NLR *101*

VICTOR SHIH: *author of* Factions and Finance in China *(2008); at* UC *San Diego*

PETER SOMERVILLE: *at University of Lincoln; works include* Understanding Community *(2016)*

FREDERIK VAN DAM: *teaches European literature at Radboud University; author of* Anthony Trollope's Late Style: Victorian Liberalism and Literary Form *(2016)*

SUSAN WATKINS

AMERICA vs CHINA

ESCALATING TENSIONS between Washington and Beijing do not yet constitute a new cold war. But they signal an important shift in US policy. From the 1990s—orchestrating China's entry into the WTO, guaranteeing its dollar assets at the peak of the financial crisis—the emphasis had been on cooperation, if backed by military might. Today, Washington is threatening to ramp up a tariff war and instructing NATO members to boycott the PRC's market-leading 5G technology. The Department of Justice has staged a spectacular international arraignment of a Chinese tech company's chief executive for dealing with Iran. The latest US National Security Strategy statement classifies China, alongside Russia, as a 'revisionist power'. America had hoped that integration into the international order would liberalize China, the NSS document explained. Instead, the PRC was trying to expand the reach of its 'state-driven economic model'. It aimed to displace the US from the Western Pacific and reorder the region to suit itself. There was self-criticism, too. As solo superpower after the Cold War, Washington had been too complacent. 'We assumed that our military superiority was guaranteed and that a democratic peace was inevitable. We believed that liberal-democratic enlargement and inclusion would fundamentally alter the nature of international relations and that competition would give way to peaceful cooperation.' Instead, a new era of 'great power competition' has dawned, involving a systemic clash 'between free and repressive visions of world order'.[1]

Though the tougher American stance has broad support across party lines, Wall Street is nervous. Robert Rubin told *New York Times* readers that China can't simply be instructed to change its economic model, although it should recognize that some consequences of its system were unacceptable to the US. Martin Wolf explained in the *Financial Times* that the right path was to manage relations with a China that would be both 'foe and friend'. But the liberal media has largely backed the new line. 'International suspicion has as much to do with the nature of China's system as with the company [Huawei] itself', stated the *Financial Times*. 'Trump has been right to press all the issues', declared the NYT. The *Economist* agreed: 'America needs to be strong'—'Trump's willingness to disrupt and offend can be effective.'[2] A lead text in the latest number of *Foreign Affairs* dials up the charges. China is seeking 'complete dominance' in the Indo-Pacific region, where it aims to be the 'unchallenged political, economic and military hegemon'. Beijing has been able to pick and choose in its support for the US-designed institutions of the global order—the UN, WTO, World Bank—and has built support for itself in regions where the US has been (relatively speaking) absent: Africa, Central Asia, Iran, Sudan, North Korea. It has been undermining the US alliance system in Asia—encouraging the Philippines to distance itself from Washington, supporting Seoul's opening to Pyongyang, backing Japan against US tariffs. Though America should hope to maintain its Asian pre-eminence through 'competitive but peaceful' means, it should brace itself for the use of military force.[3]

I

How serious are these new great-power antagonisms, and what is their logic? Unpacking the structural relations between the two is complicated not only by their mutual interdependence but by the disparities between them, both as 'friends'—financial and economic partners—and as 'foes'. These asymmetries characterize not only their size, wealth, power and political models, but their aims and objectives. In the last age of great-power competition, the protagonists were of the same genus: advanced industrial-capitalist nation-states, though expanding at uneven speeds and with unequal overseas possessions. In the present

---

[1] *National Security Strategy of the United States of America*, Washington, DC 2017, pp. 25, 27, 45–6.
[2] Editorial Board, 'Huawei will struggle to assuage Western concerns', FT, 28 January 2019; Editorial Board, 'You don't understand tariffs, man', NYT, 4 December 2018; 'China vs America', *Economist*, 18 October 2018.
[3] Oriana Skylar Mastro, 'The Stealth Superpower: How China Hid Its Global Ambitions', *Foreign Affairs*, Jan–Feb 2019.

case, both bodies are singular entities, like nothing else that has existed on Earth. One is a globe-straddling free-market superpower, the other a peasant-based Communist state that has undertaken thirty years of high-speed capitalist growth.

The Soviet Union was a singular entity, too. But the USSR was founded as a negation of the capitalist system—its opposite, Lenin said. The PRC likewise. Yet China has become the most dynamic sector of that system, yielding high returns for Atlantic capital, investing trillions in dollar assets and securing America's 'great moderation' of wages and prices with its armadas of container ships, ploughing the Pacific to stock America's shelves. The financial and economic interdependencies between them are not only asymmetrical—poor creditor, rich debtor—but operate at many different levels, which have themselves been adjusting in different directions and at different tempos, and remain at the mercy of variable currencies. Economic commentators saw the trade imbalances between the two as the greatest risk to systemic stability, before the looming financial crisis seized their attention in 2007. Since then, the value of US imports from China has risen by 57 per cent, while the PRC provides an irreplaceable market for US agricultural, aerospace and machinery products. Yet areas of symbiosis contrast with sharpening sectoral competition, not just in the US but across rich-world markets.

Domestically, the two economies provide a different set of contrasts. America's is a mature, continental capitalism whose manufacturing sector reached peak growth seventy years ago. For the last forty it has been struggling with falling profit rates, met by downward pressure on wages, offshoring and flight to the higher returns of asset speculation and overseas investment. But if its share of world GDP has shrunk since 1945 from a half to a quarter, America has strengthened its global lead in finance, cultural production and technological innovation in the digital era, itself 'Made in USA'. By comparison, China's GDP per capita is less than a seventh of the US level and its share of world output is 18 per cent. But Chinese growth has roared along at a sustained annual average of 10 per cent for three decades, only slowing in the last few years. Since the seventies, wealth production in the US has slowly shifted from rustbelt to sunbelt, with hoards of wealth accumulating in a few dozen counties. Over the same period, China has transformed itself from a rural Asian country to an ultra-modern, urbanized society.

In this spectacular case of late-comer combined development, it's not easy to distinguish the country-of-origin of the factors involved. China launched its manufacturing take-off in the nineties on tides of trade that were fast globalizing under American direction—tariffs falling, investment capital swirling, the logistics of containerization locking into place. These were preconditions for its growth. But the PRC borrowed the initial formula for its export-led model from East Asia's 'flying geese', and much early capital came from the regional Chinese diaspora, as well as Hong Kong, Taiwan and Japan. Offering cheap, biddable labour for assembly work in purpose-built Special Economic Zones, it acquired the technical know-how of modern manufacturing while sucking in export earnings. But the magnet that attracted American, Japanese and European firms to set up shop there in the 1990s was 'Made in China': a vast domestic consumer market, whose economic and cultural capacities had developed under Communist rule. Peasant literacy, an emancipated female labour force and a bureaucratic nerve system extending to every village, able to command bank lending, organize infrastructure and control capital flows—these home-grown factors, as much as its size, set China's development apart from the other 'newly industrializing countries'.

2

As political-economic entities, the two have not only been growing at different speeds but each has been changing, internally and externally, in different ways. During the Cold War, the US as world hegemon tolerated a high degree of economic protectionism in its camp. As the Communist threat receded and inter-capitalist competition intensified, Washington abandoned its self-denying ordinance and began to use its global weight to assert American national interests.[4] Nixon revoked Bretton Woods in favour of the fiat-dollar system. Reagan officials strong-armed Germany and Japan to revalue their currencies, to give US exporters an extra edge. The World Bank and IMF were used to prise open crisis-stricken economies and put their assets up for sale.

---

[4] Perry Anderson, 'Imperium', NLR 83, Sept–Oct 2013, p. 16; and *American Foreign Policy and Its Thinkers*, London and New York 2015, p. 17. Here the fit and friction between the universal-capitalist and the national-supremacist aspects of US hegemony, varying over time, are examined in detail.

These were the first inklings of a new imperial order that took full form once the US emerged as the sole superpower. It instituted a regime of 'structural reforms' that penetrated deep into the economic and political life of other states, opening them up to international flows of finance and trade. The reforms centred on the property rights of Atlantic firms and investors, operating overseas, enabling them to gain ownership of domestic assets in other countries and integrate them into global profit streams. With them, the US instituted a sea change in inter-state relations, abandoning the 'Westphalian' principle of sovereign-state jurisdiction. Sovereignty was now reconceived as a partial and conditional licence, which could be withdrawn if a state failed to comply with the liberal economic and political norms set by the US-led 'international community' and monitored by its global institutions.[5] Meanwhile, the erosion of other states' sovereignty was matched by its accumulation at the imperial centre, where the US arrogated to itself the right of regime change, with or without the consent of its allies. It embarked on a distinctively national, oil- and Israel-centric programme of warfare across the greater Middle East.

Under this new order, Washington's policy towards China was crystal-clear. The guidelines set out in its 1993 National Security Strategy have been followed unbendingly ever since. The strategic priority for the US after the Cold War was to prevent the emergence of a new superpower. It would maintain the unchallenged aerial and naval supremacy over the Pacific region that it had enjoyed since 1945. Washington would watch China closely and 'support, contain or balance' as need be. The aim was to press Beijing to implement the structural reforms spelled out by the World Bank—to open its markets fully to North Atlantic firms and investors, and guarantee their property rights. Washington hoped that socializing Chinese elites within its university system would help to produce a new layer of Yeltsins and Gorbachevs, open to the idea of replacing the CCP with a more acceptable form of rule.

Beijing has manifested no corresponding ambition to reform America's domestic system, nor to challenge head-on the new inter-state order.

---

[5] Peter Gowan, 'Neoliberal Cosmopolitanism', NLR 11, Sept–Oct 2001. The 1648 Treaty of Westphalia put an end to Europe's devastating seventeenth-century wars of religion through a mutual agreement to respect the sovereign's domestic jurisdiction.

The dual objective of the CCP has been to protect the political-economic model it had built and to upgrade China's status within the American-run international system. In contrast to the hard-boiled prose of US policy documents, public iterations of China's 'grand strategy' have been nebulous, where not negative. 'Maintain a low profile, hide brightness, do not seek leadership, but do some things', in the wisdom attributed to Deng Xiaoping. In practice, China's foreign policy has been wavering. With an eye to pleasing the Americans, it has lurched into aggressive moves against 'fraternal' regimes: the disastrous invasion of Vietnam in 1979; dispatch of Uighurs to support the American-backed Mujahideen in Afghanistan; joining the US in sanctions against North Korea. Belying its occasional fulminations against hegemonism, it cast its UNSC vote in favour of the occupation of Iraq and the bombardment of Libya.

Operating within the new globalized order, Beijing hoped to shield itself from the fate that had befallen the region's 'open markets' during the 1997 Asian crisis, when the IMF descended upon Jakarta, Bangkok and Seoul. Capital controls and a vast hoard of dollar earnings were its first lines of defence—opening up a $2 trillion trade surplus with the US, on whose consumers the Chinese export model came to depend. At the same time, the CCP leadership aimed to graduate as swiftly as possible from the export model to domestically driven growth, through a gigantic programme of internal investment. From the early 2000s, the physical reconstruction of the country—hundreds of new cities, thousands of miles of super-highways, power plants, viaducts, high-speed trains—sucked in raw materials and inputs from states across the southern hemisphere, for whom China became a major trading partner: Brazil, Argentina, Venezuela, Zambia, Sudan, Australia, Indonesia. In the process, it emerged as a world-beating builder of infrastructure, throwing up highways across Andean mountainsides and bridges between Indian Ocean islands, the contracts eased by cheap loans. The new China shone a bright light on the limits of US power, the zones that structural adjustment left undeveloped, the countries punished at Washington's whim.

3

The financial crisis brought about a watershed in US–China relations. A good part of Beijing's dollar reserves had been confidently parked in Fanny Mae and Freddie Mac. The discovery that they were now disappearing in the credit meltdown came as a shock. 'When we were elated about the rapid growth in foreign reserves, China had unconsciously fallen into a "dollar trap",' one expert put it.[6] Washington took the mortgage-makers into its conservatorship. But this was only one fire to put out. Far more dangerous was the risk to the Atlantic banking system as a whole. The Federal Reserve set in place semi-covert currency swap-lines with the central banks involved. Russia and China were excluded.

For Washington, the biggest geo-political shock came from Japan, where the opposition Democratic Party was elected in a landslide in August 2009. Its leader announced that the failure of the Iraq War and the Wall Street crash showed that the era of US-led globalization was coming to an end, and welcomed the coming age of multipolarity. Japan now recognized that the East Asian region was its basic sphere of being. It should aspire to regional currency integration—with China—as a natural extension of economic growth, with a new security framework to match. It demanded that the US shift from its enormous military and naval base at Okinawa, the southern island closer to Fujian than to Tokyo, commanding the Western Pacific and East and South China Seas. The Obama Administration mobilized its forces against the plan. By April 2010, Hatoyama had crumbled. Obama's 'pivot to Asia'—60 per cent of American firepower would be based there—was set in train.

Beijing's reaction to the crisis was two-fold. At diplomatic level, the Hu Jintao government resolved to 'diversify' its foreign policy. While Washington was still 'the key of the keys', 'surrounding areas are the first priority, developing countries are the foundation, multilateral forums are the important stage'. Meanwhile, Beijing combined an epic stimulus package with an instruction to banks to double their lending targets, the overall effect estimated at nearly 20 per cent of GDP. The central authorities specified sectors where this should be spent by regional and lower-level governments—health, education, low-income housing, digital R&D, environmental protection and so on—though much found its way into misallocation, speculative bubbles and murky loans. In the short term growth was restored through a sharp tilt towards the

---

[6] Yu Yongding, director of CASS Institute of World Economics and Politics, speaking in 2011. Cited in Jonathan Kirshner, *American Power after the Financial Crisis*, Ithaca 2014, p. 115.

SOEs and state-protected financial sector that the World Bank deplored, behind the protection of reinforced capital controls. Growing internal debts, rolled over between one state body and another, were all the more reason for China not to open its markets any further to Atlantic capital; a slowing economy, and simmering popular discontent, more grounds for political repression.

As overcapacity built up in the domestic construction sector, the Xi Jinping government gave strategic form to the project of winning contracts abroad. Announced in 2013, the Belt and Road Initiative would spread westward across Eurasia and down to Singapore, linking ports from Hambantota to Gwadar and Djibouti along the continent's southern oceans. Loans and invoices could be arranged outside the dollar system. At the same time, American observers began to report rapid Chinese advances in digital technology, facial recognition and artificial intelligence, fed by the data streams from its vast online population.

4

On one view, the PRC has been a classic example of uneven capitalist growth, driving the emergence of a new great power that was bound to cause frictions for the existing partition of the earth. But in 1914, the European great powers were so evenly matched in military and economic strength that they could fight each other into the ground for four years before one side prevailed. Today, the American imperium is so vast, so overweening in its demands, that any fast-rising power must immediately grate against it. Yet its military strength makes its overthrow impossible. Either submission or an impasse must result.

The Trump Administration has coarsened the tone of US relations with China. But Washington's policy shift from 'support' to 'balance and contain' was already under way. The rising tensions between the two are, once again, asymmetrically determined, though it remains to be seen whether Xi will prove more belligerent than his predecessors. But such is the interdependency between the two powers that many of Washington's weapons may prove double-edged. Trade has increased even as tensions have risen. Trump's tariff war already threatens to hurt domestic constituencies in the US with electoral and political weight—

farmers, bankers, aerospace and machine-tools companies—whereas the political system in the PRC can more easily batten down domestic dissatisfaction at belt-tightening generated by foreign blockades. The Federal Reserve could whisk investment capital out of China by raising interest rates, but that would plunge the US and the rest of the world back into recession. Financial sanctions, of the sort honed against Iran and Russia—and now being tested out on Huawei chief executives—have no blowback effects at home but put a strain on allies. Even Germany is resisting the latest tactics against Tehran. Sabre-rattling in the Taiwan Straits or South China Sea would rally the Chinese population behind Xi, while alarming Wall Street. American foreign policy on its present course is driving Russia, China and Iran into a *de facto* alliance.

But China's options are even more constrained. It cannot afford to dump its dollars and lacks any equivalent of America's rich-state alliance system. What it can do is to avail itself of the traditional weapon of the weak—to agree, but then do nothing. That makes the greatest likelihood a concertina pattern of drawn-out attrition—heightened periods of pressure alternating with détente, summit-level agreements interspersed with alarms and shadow boxing, sudden crises over spy planes, interventions to fan or quell revolts. The flashpoints are many.

5

Yet the medium-term direction of the Chinese state, the largest in the world, remains hard to read. This is in large part because the character of the state itself, and the economy over which it presides, are both so opaque. In this number of NLR we publish three contrasting perspectives on the relations between the two. In 'The CPC and the Ancien Régime', Peter Nolan sets out the conception of the role of market and of officialdom that informs the Xi Jinping regime's approach, drawing on the ideological resources of Confucianism. In this view, state regulation, with the CCP at its core, is essential for shaping the market to serve the population's needs. Christopher Connery's 'Ronald Coase in Beijing' tracks the reform era in the footsteps of the Chicago economist's *How China Became Capitalist* to discover instead a peculiarly Chinese version of state-enabled neo-liberal culture taking root. Finally Victor Shih, in discussion with Robert Brenner, offers a unified analysis of the role of the regime as steward of China's export-led rise, through to its present attempts to steer the debt-laden economy between the Scylla of recession and the Charybdis of capital flight.

Questions could be asked of each of them. Nolan: how close is the fit between Confucian political economy and actually existing state practice? Connery: does the sinified brand of neoliberalism that Coase applauded exhaust Chinese realities? Shih: what are the politics of the economic dilemmas with which the CCP is wrestling—what contending forces are in play, inside and outside the Party? As far as US–China tensions are concerned, each perspective has a different implication. Although, as he points out, the outcome is still an open question, the logical import of Nolan's reading would be that the fundamental alterity of the PRC's economic system will make these clashes inescapable. In Connery's case, the US will have nothing to worry about as far as capitalism is concerned, though it's right to be apprehensive on the score of economic primacy. Shih's account would imply that the very—debt-dependent—alterity of the Chinese system is the reason why the US has, in truth, little to worry about in terms of either systemic challenge or economic competition. Three different logics, then, to inform thinking on the future relations between the two powers.

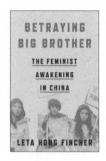
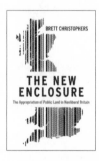

OUT NOW FROM VERSO

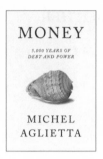
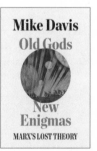

PETER NOLAN

THE CPC AND

THE ANCIEN RÉGIME

It would be impossible to read the correspondence from an Intendent of the *Ancien Régime* to both his superiors and his subordinates without being struck by how the similarity of institutions made the administrators of that era like those of our own day. They seem to reach out to each other across the chasm of the Revolution which separates them . . . Let us cease to be surprised at the marvelous ease with which centralization was re-established in France at the beginning of this century. The men of '89 had overturned the building but its foundations had stayed in the very hearts of its destroyers and, upon these foundations, were they able to rebuild it, constructing it more stoutly than it had ever been before.

Alexis de Tocqueville, *The Ancien Régime and the French Revolution*

T HE COLLAPSE OF the Soviet Union had a profound impact on China's thinking about political ideology, institutions and development.[1] The disastrous consequences for social welfare in Russia arising from the CPSU's demise reinforced Beijing's determination to resist external and internal pressure to move towards parliamentary democracy. Why did the Communist Party of the Soviet Union disintegrate while the Communist Party of China (CPC) was able to survive and strengthen its position? The dramatic divergence in the trajectories of the two Communist superpowers has been of incalculable significance for the global political economy of the twenty-first century, with effects potentially enduring far into the future.

The two regimes had a common point of departure in the political-economic system established in Russia in 1917–21. Its essential features—a monopoly of political control in the hands of the Party, state ownership of the means of production, state control over finance and trade—were devised during the extreme violence and struggle for survival of the fledgling Bolshevik regime during Russia's civil war. When it was founded in 1921, the Communist Party of China adopted fundamentally the same political structure and the same approach to economic organization. As Xi Jinping put it in 2017: 'The salvoes of the October Revolution brought Marxism-Leninism to China. In the scientific truth of Marxism-Leninism, Chinese progressives saw a solution to China's problems.'[2]

In both the USSR and China, civil war and the struggle for national survival against an invading power—respectively, Nazi Germany and Imperial Japan—reinforced the centralist, disciplinarian aspects of the Communist Party. In both countries, the period of the 'New Economic Policy'—in the early 1920s, under Lenin, and the early 1950s, under Mao—temporarily modified the approach to economic strategy, but the philosophy of the 'whole economy as a single factory', including the organization of the rural population in collective farms, was quickly reestablished as the key to economic organization on both sides of the Amur River. This 'Stalinist' economic system, alongside monolithic political control by the Party apparatus, persisted in China up to the death of Mao in 1976 and in Russia until the ascent of Gorbachev as General Secretary of the CPSU in 1985.

Polity of the tsars

However, the common features of the political-economic systems of the two Communist powers disguised profound differences in the nature of their pre-revolutionary regimes. For the CPSU, the *ancien régime* was the Russian state established from the seventeenth century onwards by the tiny Principality of Moscow through a long series of military conquests. This expansionist polity was ruled by a centralized, authoritarian government equipped with a huge army, necessary in the first instance to hold together a vast, sparsely populated and ethnically diverse territory with strong inbuilt fissiparous tendencies, and which was then tested in fierce struggles with neighbouring countries: the Great Northern Wars with the mighty Swedish state between 1700–21, the Napoleonic invasion of

---

[1] I am grateful to Dr Zhang Jin for extensive discussion of the issues raised in this paper.

[2] Xi Jinping, 'Speech at the 19th Congress of the Communist Party of China', 2017.

1812, the Crimean War against France, Britain and the Ottoman Empire in the 1850s, the Russo-Japanese War of 1904. The First World War was the last and most devastating in a long series of conflicts between Imperial Russia and its great-power rivals.

In social terms, the upper reaches of the Tsarist military and civil service were staffed by a landlord class dependent on the sovereign for the allocation and protection of its holdings. This layer had been illiterate, by and large, through to the seventeenth century, as was most of the clergy. Russia had a negligible written tradition, with a minimal place for ethical or philosophical thinking about the role of the ruling class. The Orthodox Church was reduced to the position of a subordinate branch of the state, which appointed and paid its priests and high officials. The mass of peasants, foot soldiers for the army, were virtual slaves and remained subservient even after Emancipation in 1861. Although the country possessed a highly developed internal trading system, the merchant class was kept under tight control. The Tsarist regime established state monopolies for merchants, systematically taxed their profits to support the national treasury, and took care to prevent substantial commercial cities from materializing.

While an important part of Russian culture derived from interaction with the Eastern Mediterranean and Central Asia, from Peter the Great onwards the country's rulers were above all concerned with absorbing the technologies and culture of Western Europe. This impulse was reflected in the architecture of St Petersburg, the adoption of the French language by the landholding upper classes and the orientation of the intellectual strata that emerged in the nineteenth century. This intelligentsia enthusiastically assimilated political ideas from Western Europe, and much of its literary and political activity was critical of Tsarist authoritarianism. The tension between the intelligentsia and the state would survive into the Soviet period. Capitalist industry grew between 1890 and 1914, but remained largely concentrated in St Petersburg and occupied a peripheral role in the overall political economy of Tsarism through to the eve of the Bolshevik takeover. The pre-revolutionary ruling class of landlords and military officers was preoccupied with exercising control over the Empire and the peasant masses. Its bureaucracy was relatively small. It had little understanding of the market economy and a deep sense of inferiority in relation to Western European culture.

The concept of a non-market economy based on common ownership of the means of production was central to the ideology of the Communist Party in the Soviet Union. It was implemented during the period of War Communism in 1918–21, and succeeded in throwing up a vast industrial bulwark that stopped the Nazi advance into Eurasia twenty years later.[3] However, once the CPSU leadership's faith in communism evaporated, it lost its way completely. Faced with setting a course forward in new conditions, it had no conception of what the Chinese call 'the other bank of the river'—the concrete situation it wished to attain. The only resources that Moscow's pre-revolutionary history could offer were idealized visions of Western politics and free-market economics.

Resources for the journey

At the same time, the CPC could draw upon the deep resources of the Chinese *ancien régime*. In contrast to Muscovy—little more than a wooden fortress before the fourteenth century—for millennia the densely populated, economically developed core of the state in eastern China provided a firm foundation for long periods of stable political rule, even as control over thinly settled outer territories waxed and waned. The CPC was also bolstered by the long political-philosophical tradition of the Chinese bureaucracy, whose scholar-officials were systematically inculcated with a duty to 'serve the people' and with the moral requirement placed by Mencius upon those who 'first attain understanding'.[4]

This philosophy was deeply embedded in the thinking of the traditional bureaucracy and was equally ingrained in the ideology of the CPC. Yang Changji, Mao Zedong's teacher in Changsha between 1913 and 1919 who 'made the strongest impression' on the future leader, believed fervently that scholars had a special duty to put the fate of the country above their individual desires.[5] 'Serve the people'—*wei renmin fuwu*—has echoed, as a central call of the CPC, from Mao's speech in September 1944, five years

---

[3] László Szamuely, *First Models of the Socialist Economic System: Principles and Theories*, Budapest 1974.

[4] The 4th-century BC Confucian philosopher Mencius, or Meng Zi, had posed the problem: 'I am among the first of Heaven's people to awaken. I shall awaken this people by means of the Way. If I do not awaken them, who will do so?' *Mencius*, trans. D. C. Lau, London 1970, book V, part A, section 7.

[5] Yang Changji cited the precepts of Fan Zhongyan, minister to an 11th-century Song emperor: 'Bear the hardship and bitterness before others, enjoy comfort and happiness after others' [*xian tian xia zhi you er you, hou tian xia zhi le er le*].

before the People's Republic was proclaimed, to Xi's collected addresses.[6] It need hardly be said that few, if any, bureaucrats throughout Chinese history have been able to meet the high standards of selflessness, courage and responsibility required of the ideal government official. Between 2012 and 2017, the CPC's Central Commission for Disciplinary Inspection took action against 1.4 million Party members in order to contain the rampant corruption within the Party which had spread with the growth of the 'market economy', as it is known in China—most notably in the massive property-development sector.

The idea of a non-market economy, with common ownership of property, also has ancient origins in China, going back to the words attributed to Confucius in the *Book of Rites*, itself compiled from earlier texts in the second century BC. It is clear that Confucius had in mind an ideal world, in which benevolence is the guiding principle; but the nature of property rights in such a world is open to debate.[7] Indeed, the critical passage is ambiguous: *da dao zhi xing ye, tian xia wei gong*. According to the Republican-era philosopher Feng Youlan, this sentence should be interpreted as: 'When the Great Tao was in practice, the world was common to all.'[8] His contemporary, the Japanese scholar Tsuchida Kyoson, rendered it: 'When the Great Way is realized, all the world will be in common possession.'

A generation earlier than Feng Youlan, the Utopian thinker Kang Youwei, a constitutional monarchist and leader of the 1898 Reform Movement, had proposed a similar reading of Confucius. In his *Da Tong Shu* [*Book of Great Harmony*], Kang portrayed a society in which 'all industry will be publicly controlled' and 'all commerce will revert to the control of the ministry of commerce of the government'. Economic planning would be carried out on a world scale, so that 'the evils of under- and over-production can be avoided'. In the countryside 'all land will be publicly owned and operated', while planning would extend to every detail, including work patterns, which would be executed 'like military orders'.[9]

---

[6] Mao Zedong, 'Serve the People' [8 September 1944], *Selected Readings from Mao Tse-tung*, Peking 1971; Xi Jinping, *The Governance of China*, Beijing 2014, p. 30.

[7] L. G. Thompson, 'Introduction', *The One-World Philosophy of Kang Yu-wei*, London 1958, pp. 27–9.

[8] Fung Yu-lan [Feng Youlan], *A Short History of Chinese Philosophy*, ed. Derk Bodde, New York 1948, p. 202.

[9] The *Da Tong Shu* was published in Chinese in an abbreviated form in 1913 and in full in 1935, eight years after Kang Youwei's death.

Mao was thoroughly familiar with *Da Tong Shu*. He argued that the only way to achieve the 'world of great harmony' was through a people's republic, led by the working class.[10] Many of the features of *Da Tong Shu* are similar to measures put into effect under Mao's leadership between 1956 and 1976, in the teeth of fierce opposition within the CPC. Indeed the ideas of the *ancien régime* in China, stretching back to the pre-Qin world, figure far more frequently in Mao's speeches and writings than do the ideas of Marx. *The Communist Manifesto* had a tremendous impact on him and he also made great use of Marx's writings on the Paris Commune and his *Critique of the Gotha Programme*. But apart from this, he does not appear to have made a systematic study of Marx's writings. The implementation under Mao of an economic system that virtually eliminated the market may have owed more to the radical streams in the history of Chinese thought than it did to *Capital*.

New buildings, old foundations

From the mid 1950s until the late 1970s, the main body of property in China was held in common ownership of one form or another. In December 1978, at the beginning of the reform process, the CPC took the decision to leave 'the Maoist shore' of the river—the administratively controlled economy, with common ownership of property—and cross to the other side. The nature of the other shore was left unspecified at the time. However, as China embarked on this journey, the gradual development of the 'market economy' interacted with a reintegration of the older tradition of Chinese political and ideological thought.

China's history as a state dates to the Qin Dynasty in the third century BC; its philosophical traditions go back to the Zhou Dynasty (eleventh century BC–221 BC). The *ancien régime* 'foundations' for the CPC include the long history of the Chinese bureaucracy, based on a sophisticated literary and philosophical tradition codified in the imperial examination system. Meeting the needs of the mass of the population was understood as a political-philosophical principle, and a key task for the bureaucracy was nurturing the market in order to achieve economic prosperity. This relationship was famously formulated by Guan Zhong (720–645 BC), the renowned chancellor of the State of Qi in the Spring and Autumn period of Chinese history. The text that bears his name argues that, with

---

[10] Mao Zedong, 'On the People's Democratic Dictatorship' [1949], in *Selected Readings*, 1971.

the market brought into full play, everyone could benefit; but the market alone should 'not be allowed to decide the abundance or deficiency of commodities'. There is a 'right way' to go about this, which the *Guan Zi* calls 'handling the market'.[11]

Other schools of thought existed, but views such as those expounded at the Salt and Iron Conference of 81 BC, which advocated that China should return to a Golden Age of barter in which the population 'lived contentedly and demanded little', were rarely in the mainstream of government policy. Far from eliminating the market, the state persistently sought ways to enable it to function more effectively through pragmatic and intelligent regulation—organizing a wide array of public works, including water conservation and transport infrastructure; attempting to stabilize prices of key commodities; developing famine-alleviation schemes; supporting the spread of knowledge through encyclopaedias and other written texts.

Under this system, China was a world leader in market-driven innovation for two millennia. Its inventions included the equine harness, paper and printing, advanced metallurgy through the use of the blast furnace, porcelain, tubular metal weapons, gunpowder for military purposes, the maritime compass, the sternpost rudder, watertight ship compartments, and canal-lock gates. The key components of the steam engine, the double-acting piston and the conversion of rotary to rectilinear motion—the quintessential breakthrough of the British Industrial Revolution—were developed independently in China.[12] The Chinese intelligentsia formed the core of the bureaucratic system; working within it was perfectly compatible with severe criticism of the way in which officialdom operated, even though this rarely sought the overthrow of the system itself. During this long history, the state aimed to support the economy through undertaking key functions that the market was unable to deliver; the market was always subject to regulation by the philosophically guided state.

The approach followed by the Chinese leadership since 1978 has borne a legible relationship to this tradition. From the beginning of the reform

---

[11] Guan Zhong, *The Guan Zi*, trans. by Zhai Jiangyue, 4 vols, Guangxi 2005, chapter 5, *cheng ma.*

[12] Joseph Needham, 'The Pre-natal History of the Steam Engine', in *Clerks and Craftsmen in China and the West*, Cambridge 1970.

process and 'opening up', Deng Xiaoping made clear that henceforth China should follow a pragmatic and experimental path regarding relations between state and market. The market should not be left to function without guidance, but the state should continuously 'seek the truth from the facts' in relation to their respective contributions to the economic system. In the immediate aftermath of the trauma of 4 June 1989, Jiang Zemin reiterated: 'The extent, method and scope of combination between the planned economy and regulation through the market should be constantly adjusted and perfected in accordance with the actual situation.'[13] Within the political philosophy of the *ancien régime*, this pragmatic perspective suggests that the correct way to regulate the market involves a non-ideological search for balance and interaction between the *yin* of the ethically guided state and the *yang* of market competition. The famous passage in the *Book of Rites* can be regarded as a philosophical foundation for this approach. As Wu Guozheng suggested, it can be interpreted thus: 'When the great principle prevails, the whole world is bent upon the common good.'[14]

Alternative paths

There has been fierce debate in China in recent decades on the nature of the country's history and intellectual traditions, both on their own terms and in relation to those of the West. The distinctive character of this discussion can be seen in the willingness of Chinese intellectuals, not least those within the CPC, to combine reflections on their own past with investigations into Western history and philosophy, to help clarify the outlines of 'the other shore'. In this they were following in the steps of Mao, who famously wrote: 'Use the past to serve the present, and use the foreign to serve China.' Mao's tutor, Yang Changji, was a pioneer in the effort to engage closely with Western intellectual traditions. In the work of Adam Smith, China's current leaders discerned a similar concern with state-market relations. In *The Wealth of Nations*, Smith famously analysed the contribution of the invisible hand of market competition to social and economic progress in the West. However, both there and,

---

[13] Jiang Zemin, 'Speech at the Meeting in Celebration of the 40th Anniversary of the Founding of the People's Republic of China', 29 September 1989, in Research Department of Party Literature, Central Committee of the Communist Party of China, *Major Documents of the People's Republic of China*, Beijing 1991.
[14] Wu Kuo-cheng [Wu Guozheng], *Ancient Chinese Political Thought*, Shanghai 1933, p. 299.

above all, in his *Theory of Moral Sentiments*, he also argued that, left to itself, the market produces deeply problematic outcomes in terms of inequality, the nature of work, the achievement of happiness and the ethical foundations of society.

Since 1978, this philosophy has been incorporated into the outlook of the Chinese leadership, with the goal of integrating the 'visible hand' of government regulation and the 'invisible hand' of market competition, through a process of continuous experimentation with the method of combining the 'snake' of regulation and the 'hedgehog' of market competition. There have been innumerable difficulties along the way and no doubt there will be more to come. Nevertheless, China's record during this period has been remarkable. Between 1980 and 2018, its share of global GDP rose from 2.3 to 18.5 per cent, while that of the EU shrank from 30.1 to 16.2 per cent.[15] China has nurtured a formidable group of state-owned enterprises as well as powerful non-state counterparts. The principal firms are in the process of becoming globally competitive companies, with world-leading technologies, brands and reputations. Economic growth has provided the basis for a tremendous advance in popular material and cultural welfare. The expansion of the country's physical and social infrastructure systems—transport, electricity, telecommunications, water supply and sewage—has contributed to greatly improved living standards for the mass of the population. An enormous programme of housing construction has helped provide decent homes and personal security for the hugely increased number of city-dwellers. Expanded health and education provision has made a vital contribution to mass welfare.

China's 'national rejuvenation' is intimately linked to its long history of simultaneously nurturing and regulating the market. It is not hard to see why the Chinese leadership would believe that this experience could make an important contribution towards a political philosophy of intelligent, pragmatic regulation for the global economic system, in the common interest, over the decades and even centuries ahead. The CPC's programme of reform and opening up led many Western commentators to believe that the West would dominate China in the twenty-first century. These views were reinforced when China joined the WTO in 2001, but they have proved to be an illusion. The way in which China

---

[15] IMF World Economic Outlook Database 2018.

engages with the West is still an open question. The degree to which it 'absorbs the outside world' [*xishou wailai*] as opposed to 'integrating with the outside world' [*ronghe wailai*] remains unresolved. The outcome depends not only on China but also on the West.

The radically different nature of the *anciens régimes* in China and in Russia is one key reason for the survival and prosperity of the CPC and the disintegration of the CPSU. This difference has become progressively more distinct as China has moved away from the policies of the Maoist era. In the years since 1978, the nature of the 'other bank of the river' has become increasingly clear. It is not the 'common property-ism' of '*gongchan zhuyi*'. Rather, the market plays a central role in stimulating the economy, while pragmatic state regulation, with the CPC at its core, aims to ensure that the market serves the needs of the whole population. Irrespective of whether property is privately owned, held in common by the state or by cooperatives, or under mixed ownership, it will be subject to regulation by the Party and the government in the common interest. In this view, 'groping for stones to cross the river' has gradually revealed a path of reform leading towards the other bank, which might be described as a form of *da tong zhu yi*—'great harmony-ism', or perhaps 'great commonwealth-ism'—drawing upon the age-old Chinese notion of a meritocratic bureaucracy that regulates the economic system in the interests of the whole population. China still has far to go, with huge internal and external challenges. However, China's leaders and the Chinese people have been able to see increasingly clearly the broad outlines of the 'other bank' in their collective search for a 'Way' in the midst of a turbulent world.

independent thinking from polity

The Second Coming

Franco 'Bifo' Berardi

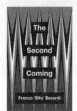

Chaos is all around us: political folly, economical delirium, ecological catastrophe, intellectual cynicism, technological simulation of life. If our world is dead, then the space is open for another to appear – a world where apocalypse can shake us out of our contemporary zombie-like existence. The second coming of communism will have nothing to do with 1917. Apocalypse has to be conceived of as a metaphor, and communism is a metaphor too: the metaphor of the possible deployment of the potentials of the mind.

January 2019
Pb 9781509534845 | £9.99

The Relevance of the Communist Manifesto

Slavoj Žižek

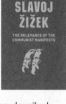

Žižek argues that, while exploitation no longer occurs the way Marx described it, it has by no means disappeared – on the contrary, the profit once generated by the exploitation of workers has been transformed into rent appropriated by the privatization of the 'general intellect'. But even if Marx's analysis can no longer be applied to our contemporary world of global capitalism without significant revision, the fundamental problem with which he was concerned, the problem of the commons in all its dimensions, remains as relevant as ever.

January 2019
Pb 9781509536115 | £9.99

Philosophical Elements of a Theory of Society

Theodor W. Adorno

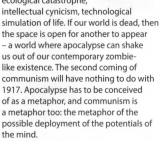

"Against the alleged waning of Adorno's radical commitments in his last years, these lectures of 1964 on the relationship between social theory and empirical research testify to his abiding Marxist loyalties. Exhorting his students to pierce the 'technological veil' of their 'administered world,' he insists on the power of class, reified consciousness, and the impoverishment of experience in the irrational totality of late capitalism."
Martin Jay, University of California, Berkeley

January 2019
Pb 9780745679488 | £17.99

Classification Struggles

General Sociology, Volume 1

Pierre Bourdieu

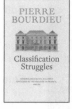

This is the first of five volumes that will be based on lectures given by Pierre Bourdieu at the Collège de France in the early 1980s. In these lectures, Bourdieu sets out to define and defend sociology as an intellectual discipline, and introduces and clarifies some of his most famous concepts. This volume focuses on the way that we classify and name the world around us, and how this gives rise to struggles that encompass race, class and gender.

January 2019
Hb 9781509513277 | £25.00

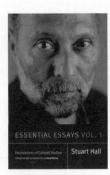
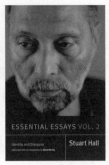
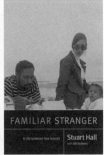

ESSENTIAL ESSAYS VOL. 1 — Foundations of Cultural Studies — Stuart Hall — Edited and with an introduction by David Morley

ESSENTIAL ESSAYS VOL. 2 — Identity and Diaspora — Stuart Hall — Edited and with an introduction by David Morley

FAMILIAR STRANGER — A Life between Two Islands — Stuart Hall — with Bill Schwarz

Stuart Hall: Selected Writings

Series Editors
CATHERINE HALL and BILL SCHWARZ

Essential Essays
STUART HALL
Edited and with an introduction by
DAVID MORLEY
Volume 1: Foundations of Cultural Studies
Volume 2: Identity and Diaspora
Also available as a set for a special price.

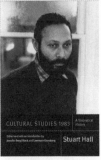

CULTURAL STUDIES 1983 — A Theoretical History — Edited and with an introduction by Jennifer Daryl Slack and Lawrence Grossberg — Stuart Hall

Familiar Stranger
A Life Between Two Islands
STUART HALL
BILL SCHWARZ, editor
US rights only

Cultural Studies 1983
A Theoretical History
STUART HALL
JENNIFER DARYL SLACK and
LAWRENCE GROSSBERG, editors

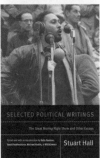

Selected Political Writings
The Great Moving Right Show and
Other Essays
STUART HALL
SALLY DAVISON, DAVID
FEATHERSTONE, MICHAEL
RUSTIN, and BILL SCHWARZ, editors
US rights only

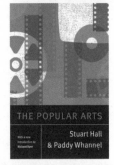

SELECTED POLITICAL WRITINGS — The Great Moving Right Show and Other Essays — Edited and with an introduction by Sally Davison, David Featherstone, Michael Rustin, & Bill Schwarz — Stuart Hall

The Popular Arts
STUART HALL and PADDY WHANNEL
With a new introduction by
RICHARD DYER

In the U.K. and Europe, contact
COMBINED ACADEMIC PUBLISHERS.
combinedacademic.co.uk

DUKE
UNIVERSITY
PRESS

    dukepress.edu

THE POPULAR ARTS — With a new introduction by Richard Dyer — Stuart Hall & Paddy Whannel

CHRISTOPHER CONNERY

RONALD COASE IN BEIJING

IN EARLY 2017, when Xi Jinping, the darling of Davos, extolled the virtues of liberalization, openness and free trade, it seemed that, whatever was happening in the West, at least the Chinese version of neo-liberalism was safe. Instead, the past two years have delivered what appear to be blatant departures from the playbook: the steady rise of *dirigisme*, and a leader (for life?) who has in recent months called for a strengthening of the state-owned enterprises (SOEs) and a recommitment to the Chinese Communist Party's version of Marxist-Leninism. Actually existing neo-liberals in China have fared poorly as well. The leadership's 2012 attacks on neo-liberal positions, along with other subversive currents—universal values, constitutional democracy, et al—cheered at the time by many on the left, have sharpened. The editors of *Yanhuang chunqiu*, the primary organ for pro-reform, pro-market, liberal intellectuals, founded in 1991, announced in 2016 that their journal would close, due to excessive government interference (publication continued under a different editorial staff). Neo-liberalism's most prominent think-tank in China, the Unirule Institute, had to suspend its popular websites and blogs in 2017. Economist Mao Yushi, Unirule's founding director and China's most celebrated neo-liberal, has been forbidden to publish, and in the summer of 2018, the Institute's Beijing headquarters were shut down, doors and windows barred.

The past year has also witnessed stepped-up surveillance of the universities, where liberal and neo-liberal ideas have long had far greater purchase than most in the West realize, with monitoring of syllabuses and class content, and with the threat of reports on faculty misconduct by the volunteer security-service informants in nearly every student body. Wang Hui and a number of other leftists once saw in the Xi regime portents of the rise of 'the people', marking a turn away from the neo-liberalism that had appeared entrenched since the mid-90s. This is a harder position to maintain today, given recent attacks on the left—the closing of websites, the arrest of feminist and worker activists, and even the threatened closure of the Beijing University Marxist Society—as well as Xi's retreat, in the face of economic headwinds, from earlier prom-ises of steadily stronger welfare protection. Still, though criticized for crudeness and over-reach, Xi has been fairly successful in promoting neo-authoritarianism at home, tightening the screws on left and right alike, while trying to present himself on the global stage as protector of free trade and a harmonious international economic order. No won-der that feminist cultural critic Dai Jinhua has described the current political-cultural landscape as being 'without coordinates'.[1]

A landscape without coordinates, though, may be one in which neo-liberalism thrives. Its core political-economic doctrine—the market as information processor and revealer of truth; competition as guarantor of optimum performance; state intervention to maintain appropriate forms of competition; a generalization of entrepreneurial values at the institutional and individual levels; and explicit or implicit anti-egalitarianism—has taken root worldwide in a variety of political contexts. Indeed, 'normative neo-liberalism'—the actualization of neo-liberal values in state policy—has arguably required Third Way or Democratic Party governance, rather than overtly market-fundamentalist parties, to thrive.[2] Neo-liberal economists and ideologues have not necessarily needed positions of political power in order for neo-liberalism to serve as a pole of attraction; few if any of China's key economic policy makers are overtly hostile to it. This intervention will argue that China's post-reform trajectory is indeed legible through a neo-liberal optic, but it is a limit case as well.

Clearly, state intervention in the economy persists in China, and its recent trajectory would appear to contradict the predictions of economists

---

[1] Dai Jinhua, 'A Cultural Landscape With No Coordinates: Contemporary Chinese Cinema', talk at the University of California Santa Cruz, 25 May 2016. A version of this talk was published as 'Zuobiao yu wenhua dixing' (Coordinates and the Cultural Landscape), *Wuyouzhixiang* (Utopia), 2 July 2017.
[2] William Davies, 'The New Neoliberalism', NLR 101, Sept–Oct 2016.

across the spectrum—from neo-liberals to industrial-policy specialists to straightforward Keynesians—of a gradually lessening role for SOEs, or at least a greater rationalization of their access to credit. Yet neo-liberalism as a doctrine has undergone numerous historical mutations—the anti-monopoly orthodoxy of the Ordo-liberals giving way to the monopoly-tolerant orthodoxy of the Chicago School, for example—coterminous with alterations in the fundamental but surprisingly fungible concept of competition. In a period like the present, with the 'Ordo-globalist' regime that Quinn Slobodian describes entering a period of (temporary?) eclipse, we might expect a proliferation of national variants of the neo-liberal dominant.[3] And of all the thinkers in the neo-liberal pantheon, perhaps the most open to multiple, variant versions of neo-liberal governance was Ronald Coase.

A singular approach

Coase did not, to my knowledge, ever identify himself as a neo-liberal, and in general avoided doctrinal orthodoxy and socio-philosophical speculation. A great admirer of Hayek and a respected member of the Mont Pèlerin Society, in the latter half of his life he became the mainstay of the law and economics orientation at the University of Chicago, teaching in the law school. His lucid and relentlessly systematic empiricism—deployed with an unassuming modesty, in contrast to many of his colleagues at Chicago—helped several of his articles to become field-defining; he was awarded the Nobel Prize for economic science in 1991. From a modest background, Coase was born in 1910 in Willesden, north London, the son of a Post Office telegraph clerk, and described himself as a socialist in his youth. He studied at the London School of Economics under Lionel Robbins, Hayek and, most influentially, the South African economist Arnold Plant, and taught there until the 1950s, his research

[3] Hong Kong-based sociologists Yin-wah Chu and Alvin So have proposed the term 'state neo-liberalism' for China, arguing for a prominent role of the state in promoting and guaranteeing a neo-liberal order. See their 'State Neoliberalism: The Chinese Road to Capitalism', in Yin-wah Chu, ed., *Chinese Capitalisms: Historical Emergence and Political Implications*, London 2010. On the mutability and internal diversity of neo-liberalism, see Philip Mirowski, *Never Let a Serious Crisis Go to Waste: How Neoliberalism Survived the Financial Meltdown*, London and New York 2014. On the global order, see Quinn Slobodian, *Globalists: The End of Empire and the Birth of Neoliberalism*, Cambridge, MA 2018.

focusing on the economics of public utilities—broadcasting and the postal services, as well as water, electricity and gas.[4]

Coase's seminal study, 'The Nature of the Firm', mentioned in his Nobel citation and published when he was only twenty-six, was the upshot of a year spent touring factories and businesses in the US in 1931–32, with the aim of exploring the different ways in which industries were organized. Instead, Coase questioned why the coordination provided by the firm's management was needed at all, if competition, acting through the price system, was supposed to supply all the coordination necessary.[5] The opening lines of the article could almost come from Marx: 'Economic theory has suffered in the past from a failure to state clearly its assumptions. Economists in building up a theory have often omitted to examine the foundations on which it was erected.'[6] Coase would remain unsurpassed among neo-liberals as a ruthless interrogator of foundations. To the question, 'Why do firms exist?', he replied that it was due to the 'transaction costs' of using the price mechanism: a firm would conduct functions in-house if this lowered the cost of obtaining the labour or services through market exchange. The concept of transaction costs opened up new fields of inquiry and shaped the New Institutional Economics, so called to distinguish it from the early 20th-century Veblen variety.

After a wartime stint at the Central Statistical Office in London, which only confirmed his scepticism about nationalized industry, Coase moved to the US in the 1950s, teaching first at Buffalo and then at the University of Virginia. In 1964 he settled at Chicago, assuming the editorship of the

---

[4] Coase addressed the Mont Pèlerin Society on the question of 'Broadcasting in a Free Society' in 1950. His first book, British Broadcasting: A Study in Monopoly, was published the same year.

[5] As Coase explained in his Nobel Prize lecture: 'The same problem presented itself to me at that time in another guise. The Russian Revolution had taken place only fourteen years earlier. We knew then very little about how planning would actually be carried out in a communist system. Lenin had said that the economic system in Russia would be run as one big factory. However, many economists in the West maintained that this was an impossibility. And yet there were factories in the West and some of them were extremely large. How did one reconcile the views expressed by economists on the role of the pricing system and the impossibility of successful central economic planning with the existence of management and of these apparently planned societies, firms, operating within our own economy?' Ronald Coase, 'The Institutional Structure of Production', 9 December 1991.

[6] Ronald Coase, 'The Nature of the Firm', Economica, November 1937. Economica was, and is, an LSE publication.

Journal of Law and Economics.[7] By then the triumph of the second article mentioned in his Nobel citation, 'The Problem of Social Cost' (1961), had enshrined his reputation. Arguing, like a lawyer, from actual cases, Coase provided a rebuttal of the prevailing view, formulated in Arthur Pigou's *Economics of Welfare* (1920), that government action was required to restrain businesses whose actions created 'negative externalities', with harmful effects on others. Coase claimed instead that negotiations between the two parties would lead to a settlement maximizing wealth, irrespective of the rights involved. 'The Problem of Social Cost' became one of the most cited articles in the discipline of economics, opening the way for US neo-liberalism's radical anti-regulatory agenda and 'out-Chicagoing Chicago'.[8]

It is thus no surprise to find in Coase, anti-dogmatist and lifelong opponent of 'blackboard economics', one of Chinese capitalism's strongest defenders. Though he himself never went to China, his work became known there in the mid-80s and his influence has remained strong ever since.[9] He was the guiding intellectual force behind the development of the Chinese version of Institutional Economics—thought by its practitioners to have particular relevance to PRC conditions, due to the wide variety of 'institutions' directly involved with the economy—and nearly all Chinese institutional economists would consider themselves Coasian. (Coase himself rejected the term 'Coasian economics', preferring that it be called 'correct economics'.) Over the 1990s and into this century, when he himself had turned ninety, Coase hosted a series of prominent Chinese economists in Chicago on research visits, as post-docs and as conference participants, and he maintained close relations with those on the neo-liberal spectrum. Steven Cheung (known in standard Chinese as Zhang Wuchang), University of Chicago post-doctoral research scholar, later at the University of Hong Kong, was particularly close to Coase, and became one of the most widely read and most

---

[7] Coase outlined his method as editor of the journal in the autobiographical note he supplied to the Nobel committee: 'I encouraged economists and lawyers to write about the way in which actual markets operated and about how governments actually perform in regulating or undertaking economic activities.'

[8] William Davies, *The Limits of Neoliberalism: Authority, Sovereignty and the Logic of Competition*, London 2015, pp. 51–4, 84–5.

[9] See Zhang Shuchang and Sheng Hong, eds, *Kesi yu Zhongguo: yiwei jingjixue dashi de Zhongguo yingxiangli* [*Coase and China: A Great Economist's Influence in China*], Beijing 2013; Steven Cohn, *Competing Economic Paradigms in China: The Co-Evolution of Economic Events, Economic Theory and Economics Education, 1976–2016*, New York 2017.

influential economists in China. Cheung's 1982 pamphlet, *Will China Go Capitalist?*, published by the London-based neo-liberal Institute for Economic Affairs, suggested a tentative yes, provided that China established a regime of property rights.

Thirty years later, Coase's *How China Became Capitalist*, co-authored with his research assistant Ning Wang, answered Cheung's question with a resounding affirmative.[10] It is an accounting of China's capitalist transformation within the parameters of Coase's neo-liberal political-economic rationality and a Hayekian episteme. A Chinese translation with the title, *Biange Zhongguo: Shichang jingjide Zhongguozhi lu* [*China in Transformation: The Chinese Road to a Market Economy*] was published in 2013. 'Capitalism', throughout the Chinese version, was translated as *shichang jingji*, or 'market economy', while 'socialism', when used in a pejorative sense, was translated as *jihua jingji*, or 'planned economy'; the few references in the original to the 1989 Tiananmen movement were eliminated. Otherwise the translation was accurate and thorough. *China in Transformation* was very successful in China, possibly because readers could find in its narrative of capitalist development both admiration for Chinese particularism and hope for continued future prosperity, with none of the typical warnings that a bright economic future would depend on adopting Western political norms. There was little of the social, nothing of class, and very little of the subjective in the book; its focus was largely on macroeconomic and industrial policy, framed by the familiar neo-liberal critique of planning or 'guiding ideas'. It did, however, render the course of reform wholly legible within a neo-liberal optic, claiming China for neo-liberalism in a Chinese way, by 'seeking truth from facts'. Through Coase and Wang's eyes, we may see indications that neo-liberalism has indeed sunken deep its roots in China.

Tigers and stones

Two Chinese proverbs dominate the homiletic register of reform discourse: 'crossing the river by feeling the stones' (*mozhe shitou guo he*)

---

[10] Ronald Coase and Ning Wang, *How China Became Capitalist*, London and New York 2012. Henceforth, HCBC. Coase explains in the preface that the pair began work on the book in 2008, when Coase was a mere 97; Wang 'provided information about events in China and their interpretation', the two authors then 'collaborated fully in discussing their significance', correcting errors and realigning arguments. The book appeared when Coase was 101; he died the following year.

and 'when riding the tiger it's hard to get off' (*qi hu nan xia*). 'Riding the tiger', used primarily outside official discourse, suggests a lack of total control: the tiger of capitalism will go where it chooses.[11] 'Feeling the stones', quoted often by early reformers including Deng Xiaoping and the 'conservative' Chen Yun, is a 'folk simile' known as *xiehouyu* in Chinese: a two-part vehicle-tenor proverb whose second part is unstated, though understood. The standard association with 'crossing the river' is 'steady and stable' (*wenwendangdang*), emphasizing the stability of the stone on which one rests, rather than, as some later usages would have it, the uncertain location of the stone to come.

Coase and Wang write in their preface that 'the series of events that led China to become capitalist was not programmed and the final result was entirely unexpected', making Chinese capitalism a pertinent illustration of 'what Hayek has called "the unintended consequences of human action"'.[12] Readers of Hayek will know, of course, that the intended consequences of human action—planning—are to be avoided, since no human intelligence could equal the superior calculation of the market. There is thus in Coase and Wang's version of the turn to capitalism no Chinese civilizational essence—as in Robert Bellah or Ambrose King's claim for affinities between Confucianism and a Tawneyan Protestantism—awaiting the dissolution of socialist shackles in order to re-emerge. Nor is it a Western imposition, or a surrender to a superior economic order. In their telling, the course of reform in China is a recapitulation of the neo-liberal episteme: its unexpectedness and unprogrammed character were its guarantees, and the flexibility and adaptability of the leadership, rather than its direction, were decisive.

How China Became Capitalist views the reform process largely 'from a Hayekian perspective, which stresses the growth of knowledge as the ultimate force driving economic change', meaning, of course, the knowledge that results from market competition.[13] Coase and Wang's narrative differs from mainstream accounts only in emphasis, as we will see below. On a question that divides some scholars—whether and to what extent the course of reform was directed by the state or primarily

---

[11] *Stricto sensu*, the original proverb is more commonly understood as 'in the midst of a risky and consequential undertaking, one must persevere to the very end'.

[12] HCBC, p. x.

[13] See the summary in Ronald Coase and Ning Wang, 'How China Became Capitalist', *Cato Policy Report*, Jan–Feb 2013.

emerged 'from below'—they see truth in both positions. There is little effort, as one would expect, to link Chinese developments with mutations in global capitalism or its regional dynamics. Structural conditions that facilitated competition and experimentation, the knowledge thereby produced, and the gradual expansion of market logic and market price, were the key determinants.

In their view, a structural precondition for the reforms was Mao-era decentralization, first aired in Mao's 1956 speech 'On The Ten Major Relationships', a text published only during the reform period in an effort to buttress reformers' claims for a Maoist pedigree. Decentralization was made policy in 1957 and implemented in 1958, putting significant powers over economic planning and administration in the hands of local and provincial authorities. This decentralization, which continued into the 1960s, had fiscal and military rationales, but these were not important. Given the dominance of political mobilization during the pre-1978 period, which was itself tied to Mao's charisma, Mao was able to influence local authorities directly, without needing the mediation of the Beijing bureaucracy, thus preserving an important space for central authority within a decentered structure.

One negative consequence of the famine that ended the Great Leap Forward—when local officials' zeal to meet Mao's directives led to information distortions, with tragic results—was that decentralization was discredited, and centralized planning regained authority. Coase and Wang conclude:

> A point stressed by Hayek, the far-reaching implications of which have yet to be fully recognized, is that the most critical advantage of a market lies less in its allocative efficiency, and more in its free flow of information. But the flow of information would not make much sense, indeed it would seem wasteful, if the problem that it helps to solve is not recognized. A market economy assumes two deep epistemic commitments: acknowledgement of ignorance and tolerance of uncertainty. It was hard for a defiant Mao and a triumphant Chinese Communist Party to accept either, even in the aftermath of the Great Leap Forward.[14]

The right kind of decentralization would thus allow focused application of local knowledge, experimentation and an inter-regional competition

---

[14] HCBC, p. 18.

that would generate more information. Ideology and politics stymied this capacity in the Mao years, but an organizational orientation toward decentralization was established, and this was able to function closer to Hayekian norms in years to follow.

Knowledge and profit

The journal *Lilun Dongtai* [*Theoretical Trends*], founded by Hu Yaobang in June 1977, was intended, claim Coase and Wang, to 'solicit articles to question and criticize the ossified socialist doctrines and Mao's radical policies, which still had a firm grip on the minds of the people'.[15] Debate and discussion—what Coase had called in an earlier article 'the market in ideas'—are seen as generative of knowledge in their model, and throughout the book they regard the presence of market-sceptical 'conservatives' not as threats or obstructions but as potential contributors to the accumulation of knowledge. 'Practice is the Only Criterion for Testing Truth' appeared in the journal in 1978, and it was widely understood as the definitive attack on Mao's ideological authority, overturning the 'Two Whatevers'—'We will resolutely uphold whatever policy decisions Chairman Mao made, and unswervingly follow whatever instructions Chairman Mao gave'—that dominated the immediate post-Mao period.

The first five-year plan after Mao's death, emphasizing capital-intensive heavy industry at a time of capital shortage, registered significant increases in grain and steel production. Proto-market innovations such as monetary incentives, piece rates and the beginnings of enterprise reform appeared under the aegis of 'socialist modernization', a term which had replaced class struggle and other more explicitly political determinants. Coase and Wang make much of the Third Plenum Communiqué of 1978, which neither mentioned the market nor provided a clear policy direction, but which nevertheless seemed in accordance with a Hayekian epistemological trend:

> It was actually quite fortunate that the Communiqué did not prescribe any specific measures, with the exception of agriculture. Given how poorly informed the Chinese leaders were at the time, any prescriptions would probably have done more harm than good. But now the Chinese

---

[15] HCBC, p. 25.

government was committed to a pragmatic approach, willing to subject everything to the test of practice, and eager to try anything that facilitated 'the growth of productive forces'. China may have been poorly equipped for a market revolution, but it was certainly mentally prepared.[16]

As reform built up steam in 1978 and 1979, a key factor for Coase and Wang, and one they find relatively neglected in other accounts, is enterprise reform. Consisting largely of horizontal consolidation, greater enterprise autonomy and managerial responsibility, enterprise reform had been advocated in the 1950s by Sun Yefang and Gu Zhun, mainstream economists in the early PRC, later disgraced as rightists but rehabilitated after Mao's death. Enterprise reform as then conceived was well within the purview of socialist economics. Coase and Wang want to demonstrate, though, that Chinese reformers soon learned that without price reform, and the information delivered to firms through the operation of prices, enterprise reform would likely fail, as it did in the early 1980s—at which point many voices arose, foremost among them the pro-market though 'conservative' economist Xue Muqiao, arguing for deepened price reform. The emphasis Coase and Wang place on these early failures reflects a conviction that enterprise reform, once embraced as a concept, must eventually result in price reform and an increased role for the market.

The more significant early reforms in leading to the market economy were, in their estimation, the 'four marginal revolutions': small private businesses in the cities, household farming, the Township-Village Enterprises (TVEs), and the Special Economic Zones (SEZs). Coase and Wang's version of these developments is similar to other mainstream narratives. Teiwes and Sun, among others, have recently made a convincing case for the top-down nature of agricultural de-collectivization, and its roots in fiscal crisis.[17] Although Coase and Wang claim agricultural de-collectivization as a bottom-up process, they are throughout the book supportive of state-directed reforms as long as they are pro-market, so the new interpretation would leave the centre of their analysis intact. The real fruits of the marginal revolutions, in their view, were growth in knowledge, growth in organizational diversity, a far greater role for

---

[16] HCBC, p. 40.
[17] Frederick Teiwes and Warren Sun, *Paradoxes of Post-Mao Rural Reform: Initial Steps Toward a New Chinese Countryside, 1976–1981*, New York 2016.

competition and a rise in general economic consciousness. Yuan Geng, the entrepreneur who in 1979 set up the Shekou Industrial Park, later incorporated into the Shenzhen SEZ, chose as a motto for his enterprise 'Time is money, efficiency is life' (*shijian jiushi jinqian, xiaolü jiushi sheng-ming*). For the Chinese, 'time is money' is associated with Shenzhen, not Benjamin Franklin, and this unfortunate bit of common sense did indeed begin at the margins.

The 1980s—the 'bird in the cage' phase, with macro-economic policy subject to state planning and the bird of the economy free within those bounds—saw political challenges to further marketization in 1982 and 1983. Challenges, for Coase and Wang, increase aggregate knowledge, so this was on the whole a salutary development. The 1980s also saw the rapid growth of economics as discipline and discourse. Economic policy makers were deeply engaged with Western and Eastern European economists, all pro-market thinkers of one stripe or another. A development that hastened the path to price reform, the 'dual track' pricing system—set prices within state quotas and market prices for production outside the quotas—was influenced by economics graduate student Zhang Weiying, who would later become one of China's most prominent neo-liberals. Price reform was badly timed, however, creating the volatility, inflation and austerity policies that contributed to social unrest all over the country in the second half of the 1980s, culminating in the Tiananmen massacre. Despite the decade's grim end, Coase and Wang find much to like about the politics of those years, especially the renewed participation of intellectuals in public life, universities and think-tanks, and the rebuilding of the legal system. They refer to the latter achievement not as the rule of law but as rule *by* law, 'an attempt to structure and regulate the hierarchy of power relations within the maze of Chinese politics'.[18]

Cognitive shifts

The 1980s was also a decade of 'new ideas'. Although mainstream economics focuses on competing interests rather than competing ideas, Coase and Wang write that clashes of ideas 'have not received their due attention' in the field. Ideas, embodied in institutions, become the basis for identity: 'a profound cognitive change takes place at the individual

---

[18] HCBC, p. 102.

and societal level when an institution that was adopted for its expected pragmatic function assumes a status role, coming to define our individual and collective identity.' The PRC, they note approvingly, always took ideas seriously, and the power of the idea of 'socialism' was a strong inhibition on the development of a market economy. But socialism, under the influence of post-1978 pragmatism, 'had been restored to what political ideologies should always be: a working tool rather than a non-negotiable goal.' Socialism could now be subjected to empirical testing and judged according to its performance.[19] The market economy was also an idea that needed promotion. Efforts to construct *homo economicus* in the 1980s and 90s commonly used the language of revolution, exhorting those apprehensive about the market to 'liberate the mind'.[20] 'Ideas', though, have a particular status in Coase and Wang's world. A chief benefit of the 'pragmatic turn' for Coase and Wang, in a process that Wang Hui has described as 'depoliticization', was its deliverance of ideas to the judgement of the market, which was also a process whereby market values—competition, efficiency, etc—would become the leading ideas, and sources of new identity.[21]

The post-Tiananmen retrenchment gave temporary strength to anti-market elements in the leadership, but after Deng Xiaoping's 1992 Southern Tour, the 'capitalism with Chinese characteristics' with which we are all now familiar quickly emerged, and became fully consolidated by the time of China's 2001 WTO accession. Coase and Wang credit ideological, policy and micro-environmental structural factors. Ideologically, Deng Xiaoping's re-definition of Marxist orthodoxy—the development of the productive forces was the essence of socialism; any policy that served the development of productive forces was *de facto* in accordance with socialism—removed any political or ideological barriers to market development. At the Fourteenth Party Congress in 1992, the development of the market economy was recognized as the ultimate goal of reform, and every Party Congress since then has affirmed the centrality of the market. Serious concern with ideological content at the CCP leadership level was over. Truth would henceforward be measurable, in GDP growth rates, income and poverty statistics, inflation statistics,

---

[19] HCBC, pp. 97–8.

[20] Joseph Fewsmith, *China Since Tiananmen: The Politics of Transition*, 2nd edition, Cambridge 2008, pp. 68–72.

[21] Wang Hui, 'Depoliticized Politics, from East to West', NLR 41, September–October 2006.

price, numbers of patents, et cetera. Succeeding leaders would propose ideological programmes of invariant vapidity: 'the three represents', the 'socialist harmonious society' and the 'Chinese dream'. As for communism, in 1978, Vice Premier Wang Zhen had visited the UK and, impressed by its prosperity and wage levels, is quoted as saying that 'Britain would simply be our model of a communist society if it were ruled by a communist party.'[22]

Price reform emerged gradually but decisively: by 1995, 78 per cent of goods and services were traded at market prices, and the black market was mostly a thing of the past. The tax reforms of 1994, which simplified and regularized taxes and eliminated the practice of individual-firm negotiated tax rates, provided an impetus for the further dismantling of the managerial contract system, which had contributed to the SOEs' isolation from market forces. The elimination of the product tax weakened incentives for local governments to take intra-provincial protectionist measures, thus strengthening the national market, and adding another arena of competition. Tax reform, Coase and Wang argue,

> turned out to have far-reaching effects, transforming regional economic dynamics from chaotic fiefdoms into a sustainable and efficient competition. Now, local governments competed against each other to attract investment by improving their infrastructure and business environment. Regional competition has been primarily responsible for China's remarkable economic dynamics since the mid-1990s.[23]

Finally, enterprise reform for SOEs was pursued in earnest through privatization, the use of IPOs to fund SOEs and uniform assets supervision. The 'iron rice bowl' tying employees and employers together was broken through unemployment insurance and the privatization of housing. Unlike many critics of CCP economic policy, Coase and Wang were not focused on the existence of the SOEs. If they had undergone enterprise reform—if they operated competitively and efficiently—their ownership was not much of a concern.

Coase and Wang follow Steven Cheung in emphasizing the importance of competition between counties (*xian*) as a primary driver of market reform. They return to Coase's seminal article, 'The Nature of the Firm', to posit the necessity of open markets—both product and factor

---

[22] HCBC, pp. 155–6.   [23] HCBC, p. 129.

markets—for a properly performing firm. Although the development of a functioning factor market lagged in the transition from a planned to a market economy, they argue that this was overcome by competition between counties in attracting firms to their newly constructed industrial parks:

> The transformation of factors into goods and services takes place within a structure of production in which factors are organized and coordinated by various arrangements, including the impersonal pricing mechanism, contracts and non-contractual personal relations. In this vast and still poorly understood arena, organization is critical. Organization was considered by Alfred Marshall to be a 'distinct agent of production'. But underdeveloped economies are characteristically defined by a want of organization. Indeed, organization is often in shorter supply than capital investment. In China, this vacuum was filled up by local governments, which still have enormous power to mobilize resources.[24]

Coase and Wang answer critics who would point to the resulting over-capacity, low physical-capital utilization rates, duplicate investment and impaired comparative advantage by drawing attention to the development of human capital and the spread of manufacturing and organizational technology that arose from inter-regional competition. Competition, they remind us, doesn't only take place over investment, but over ideas for economic development. Failure, being localized, is rarely disruptive. And since local officials' promotions are based on economic performance, there are more incentives to administer jurisdictions along enterprise lines.

Market in ideas

Premier Wen Jiabao was an admiring reader of Adam Smith, both *The Wealth of Nations* and *The Theory of Moral Sentiments*, and Coase and Wang appreciate the attention paid to the latter book in China. Without an idea like Smithian justice, they suggest—equal application of and equal protection under law—the inequality natural to and unavoidable in a capitalist economy would come at too great a cost. They would probably view Xi Jinping's ongoing crackdown on corruption in this Smithian light. *How China Became Capitalist* concludes with an extended critique of the absence of a market in ideas, which appears in its entirety in the

---

[24] HCBC, p. 142.

Chinese translation. Their critique of China's controls on free speech points to the familiar bad consequences: lack of innovation and creativity, inability of Chinese manufacturers to establish globally recognized 'brands', insufficient development of human potential, et cetera. But it is clear throughout that the testing ground for 'ideas' is and must be the market:

> Moreover, the market for ideas drives the market for goods and services in a fundamental way. As the market for goods operates under the assumption of consumer sovereignty, it is the market for ideas that directly shapes consumer wants, crucially determines what kind of consumers (as well as entrepreneurs, politicians and lawyers) we find in the economy, their characters and values, and thus ultimately decides what the market for goods is and how effectively it works.[25]

In a 1974 article, Coase had argued against the distinction between ideas and goods, and questioned why laissez-faire was deemed necessary in the realm of ideas while regulation was acceptable in the market for goods. From the vantage point of the market, in Coase's view, there is not much difference between 'ideas' and 'goods'.[26]

'Ideas' shaping consumer values, *contra* Coase's worry above, are not in short supply in China. What kind of pluralism, then, do Coase and Wang really want? They expressly do not link the market in ideas to a particular political form such as multi-party democracy. Neo-liberals have rarely been concerned with the rights of expression of social movements, labour unions, parties or other political collectivities. A 2013 Harvard study of social-media censorship in China made clear that the targets were not anti-government or anti-party sentiments, but those forms of speech that could lead to collective action, hardly a concern for Coase and Wang.[27] In their telling, something akin to the market in ideas existed in the 1980s and the early 90s, with beneficial consequences. If that experience is a model, then we might conclude that what the market for ideas needs most are more ideas about markets.

---

[25] HCBC, p. 194.
[26] Ronald Coase, 'The Market for Goods and the Market for Ideas', *American Economic Review*, vol. 64, no. 2, May 1974.
[27] Garry King, Jennifer Pan and Margaret Roberts, 'How Censorship in China Allows Government Criticism but Silences Collective Expression', *American Political Science Review*, vol. 107, no. 2, May 2013, pp. 326–43.

The current regime remains committed to its monopoly on the 'leading ideas', which seem to be selected for their vacuity. At the popular level, the reigning common sense—that stratum of ideas determining 'what kind of consumers we find in the economy'—is thoroughly economistic, and this must be counted as one of Chinese neo-liberalism's significant achievements. As Mirowski has pointed out, one of neo-liberalism's political modalities has been its ability to present itself as an anti-systemic, liberatory outside force. Markets can always be further opened, rights of ownership further extended, entrepreneurial activity further deregulated. Neo-liberal reason can thus function simultaneously as hegemonic common sense and liberatory outside, and this holds as true in China as elsewhere.

In Wang and Coase's interpretation of the two-decades-long emergence of capitalism, the knowledge formed through policy-makers' ignorance and flexibility in conjunction with market competition proved robust enough to consolidate and reproduce the new economy. But the capitalism that emerged in China—organically, in Coase and Wang's version—took place in the context of a global neo-liberalism with deep disciplinary roots in the fields of economics and law, and a distinctive political-economic rationality. This global context would shape the re-foundation of the discipline of economics in the Chinese academy, in think-tanks and in government policy, as well as the formation of *homo economicus* at the social and subjective levels.

Departmental politics

As if in response to Coase's call for a market in ideas, Beijing University scheduled a public debate in November 2016 between Coase disciple Zhang Weiying, former dean of the university's Guanghua School of Management, and Justin Yifu Lin, former chief economist for the World Bank. Both currently have faculty positions at Beijing University. The *Economist* announced the event with characteristic hyperbole:

> Perhaps the most famous debate in the history of economics was that between John Maynard Keynes and Friedrich Hayek—a clash over the benefits and perils of government intervention that exploded in the 1930s and still reverberates today. It has echoed around Chinese lecture halls in recent months. Justin Lin, a former chief economist of the World Bank, who leans to Keynesian faith in public spending, has squared off against

Zhang Weiying, a self-professed Hayekian who doubts bureaucrats can ever beat the free market.[28]

The event itself was anti-climactic, and more than a few commentators pointed out how much the two overlapped. Lin's position has always been that industrial policy is necessary for a certain phase of development, until more purely market forces can take over. Their proximity notwithstanding, this debate represents more or less the full spectrum of positions in the economics discipline in China today. University economics departments have similar sub-disciplinary compositions to those elsewhere in the world, and no one would find it odd to see, say, a public-choice economist writing for a state organ such as the *People's Daily*. Marxist political economists are mostly confined to departments of Marxism-Leninism, where the focus of political-economic scholarship is historical or theoretical, not policy-oriented. I suspect that there are more Marxists in UK economics departments than in their PRC counterparts. How Chinese economics departments became capitalist is an important part of the story.[29]

In 1980 a group including reform economist Xue Muqiao produced a document for official consumption concretely outlining the direction of reform—enterprise reorganization according to economic efficiency, commodity production, a role for the market along with the plan and further economic decentralization. Vice Chairman Li Xiannian, formerly Chairman Hua Guofeng's chief economic advisor, responded: 'I've read this twice and I don't understand it.'[30] This anecdote is commonly cited by historians as an indication of the parlous state of economic knowledge and of the discipline of economics, as the reform period began. Pre-Cultural Revolution economics was dominated by parameters set in Soviet economics and theory, the latter mostly around the question of value and to what extent it applied under socialism. Most senior

---

[28] 'China's Industrial Policy: Plan vs. Market', *Economist*, 5 November 2016.

[29] The most exhaustive treatment of this, from a left perspective, is Cohn, *Competing Economic Paradigms in China*. See also essays in Ying Ma and Hans-Michael Trautwein, eds, *Thoughts on Economic Development in China*, New York 2013. For a treatment of pre- and post-revolutionary Chinese Marxist economic engagement with neo-liberal economics, see Rebecca Karl, *The Magic of Concepts: History and the Economic in Twentieth-Century China*, Durham, NC 2017.

[30] This is widely reported: Liu Hong, *Bashiniandai: Zhongguo jingjixuerende guangrong yu mengxiang*, [*The 1980s and Chinese Economists*], Guilin 2010, pp. 58–9.

economists of all stripes were persecuted in the Cultural Revolution. The discipline's reconstruction began, at the outset of the reform period, at great speed and in a distinctive political environment. As Oxford economist Cyril Lin wrote in 1981, 'whereas in East Europe and the Soviet Union there exists a glut of theory and reform proposals chasing leaderships that are unwilling or unable to initiate fundamental reforms, China, in contrast, has a leadership which is impatient for reforms but which lacks the necessary theory and blueprints.'[31]

The rise of theory and blueprints was rapid. Economics, and economic discourse in general, came raging back. Reformer Xue Muqiao's 1979 *Research on Questions About China's Socialist Economy* sold 10 million copies, a record for a social-science publication only exceeded by obligatory sales of the works of Mao and subsequent leaders. The book attacked rigid 'Stalinist' planning and blamed leftism for a range of economic problems. It advocated decentralization, flexibility in distribution, a greater role for small individual enterprises and an overall emphasis on 'forces of production' over 'relations of production'.[32] The popularity of a book with 'economics' in its title is as significant as the book's content, given that five years earlier, 'economism' was still a term of opprobrium. Never again. Shortly after the World Bank approved China's request to rejoin it in 1980, a team of economists arrived in the country to complete the obligatory World Bank report. Over a thousand pages long, *China: Socialist Economic Development* was published in 1981. The Chinese translation was made mandatory reading in government units and economics departments, and was sold to the public at large at a subsidized price. The appearance of the report was hugely influential, setting a standard for economic reports from state institutions.

Putting economics in command

Steven Cohn's *Competing Economic Paradigms in China* and Julian Gewirtz's *Unlikely Partners* (2017) describe in detail how both the

---

[31] Cyril Chihren Lin, 'The Reinstatement of Economics in China Today', *China Quarterly*, vol. 85, March 1981, p. 4.
[32] Xue Muqiao, *Zhongguo shehuizhuyi jingji yanjiu*, Beijing 1979. In 1998, the Economics Research Institute of the Chinese Academy of Social Sciences, in conjunction with the Guangdong Jingji chubanshe, republished the book in a series of the ten most important economics texts influencing 'the new China', ranging from texts by 1950s-era economists Wang Ya'nan and Sun Yefang, to the early work of Wu Jinglian, probably the reform era's foremost economist.

discipline of economics and economic policy were refashioned from the late 1970s and through the 80s under the protection of Deng Xiaoping, with the guidance of both younger economists and those market- and reform-minded economic thinkers who had returned to work after being persecuted as rightists in the 50s and during the Cultural Revolution.[33] There were nearly continuous state-sponsored visits to Western Europe, the US, Eastern Europe and the developing world. Over the course of the 1980s, scores of students went to the US and the UK for graduate work in economics. The Chinese Academy of Social Sciences, established in 1977 and the *de facto* reform think-tank, hosted a stream of foreign economists, beginning in 1979 with the influential series of lectures by Oxford economist Włodzimierz Brus, a Polish exile considered the foremost theorist of market socialism. Brus, to a receptive audience, was a hard advocate of enterprise autonomy and of a strong role for market forces within a state-guided economy.

The Ford Foundation and the American Economic Association were key players in the establishment of the discipline. Much of the AEA work was headed by Princeton Economics professor Gregory Chow, who had studied under Milton Friedman at Chicago. Friedman himself was invited to China to give a series of lectures in 1980. Although *Freedom to Choose* had just been published, it is not clear that anyone in China knew of his affiliation with neo-liberalism, a word whose Chinese equivalent was rarely encountered until the 1990s.[34] Friedman's expertise on price, as well as his anti-inflationary fundamentalism, was a key attraction for his Chinese hosts, who struggled with inflation throughout the 1980s. Friedman himself was not initially sanguine about Chinese prospects, although long years of adulation finally tempered his dyspepsia. Price reform was high on the reformers' agenda, and Czech economist Ota Šik, who had an almost Hayekian conviction about the unsurpassability of price as information mechanism, became an influential favorite. Šik's emphasis on the 'socialist market' and the state's role as coordinator of the 'macro-distribution plan' was crucial in legitimating radical price reform within a system that persisted in calling itself socialist.[35]

---

[33] Julian Gewirtz, *Unlikely Partners: Chinese Reformers, Western Economists and the Making of Global China*, Cambridge, MA 2017. The story is also told in a more China-centred way in Liu Hong, *Bashiniandai*. For a more encyclopaedic description of 1980s economic thought organized according to topic, rather than school of thought, see Robert Hsu, *Economic Theories in China 1979–1988*, Cambridge 1991.
[34] Gewirtz, *Unlikely Partners*, pp. 83 ff.
[35] Gewirtz, *Unlikely Partners*, pp. 88–95; Liu, *Bashiniandai*, pp. 289–99.

Their insistence on the need for such reform was an important factor in the 1984 victory of the reformers over advocates of central planning, which set in motion the gradual and inexorable disappearance of non-market prices.[36]

To provide forms of management adequate to the transformed economy, the first MBA programmes—one US and one European joint venture—began in 1984. By 2000 there were over sixty, all with Western-derived curricula. Economics and management grew steadily in universities, and over the 1990s the term 'Western economics' was replaced by 'modern economics', even though most of the university textbooks were translations of US texts. By 2007 there were almost 1 million economics majors in universities, and over 3.5 million in management, representing over a quarter of Chinese university students.[37]

A defining event in advancing reform-era economic policy, stressed in both Gewirtz and Liu, was the September 1985 World Bank-sponsored conference on the ss *Bashan*, held during a week-long cruise on the Yangzi River through the Three Gorges, later to be flooded by the world's largest hydroelectric dam. The conference, ordered by Premier Zhao Ziyang and organized by Edwin Lim of the World Bank, Wu Jinglian and other senior Chinese economists, included such non-Chinese participants as James Tobin, Leroy Taylor, Alexander Caincross and János Kornai. Tobin surprised Chinese economists in his acknowledgment of a significant role for macroeconomic management, a term whose Chinese equivalent was invented during the cruise.[38] Tobin's ability to look at a few pages of data and immediately suggest macroeconomic policy correctives gave his Chinese hosts a glimpse of analytical power of a kind they had never seen before, and of an intelligence they hoped to develop in policy circles.[39] Kornai's *Economics of Shortage*, with its

---

[36] The standard account of the emergence and consolidation of market mechanisms remains Barry Naughton, *Growing Out of the Plan: Chinese Economic Reform 1978–1993*, Cambridge 1996.

[37] Haiyun Zhao, 'Economics Education in China', *International Journal of Pluralism and Economics Education*, vol. 1, no. 4, 2010, pp. 303–16.

[38] *Hongguan tiaozheng* (macroeconomic adjustment) was deemed too weak; *hongguan kongzhi* (macroeconomic control) was too redolent of central state planning; the neologism was *hongguan tiaokong*, the latter word a calque of 'adjustment' and 'control': Gewirtz, *Unlikely Partners*, p. 146.

[39] Gewirtz, *Unlikely Partners*, p. 145.

emphasis on the 'investment hunger' he claimed was common to all socialist societies, was thought highly relevant to China, and the *Bashan* cruise was the beginning of his long relationship with China. Kornai softened his anti-communism for his Chinese audience: in contrast to the positions he took in the Eastern European context, Kornai was one of several advocates of gradualism. He was highly persuasive in advocating 'price responsiveness' as the measure of an enterprise's success under macroeconomic management.

Milton Friedman returned to China in 1988, in the company of Steven Cheung for much of the visit, and his stay included a widely publicized audience with Premier Zhao.[40] Friedman was uncompromising in his advocacy of a completely unfettered market: a strong pole of attraction for common sense, including at the highest levels. In the economic-policy discussions of 1986–87, some officials called for workers' self-management as one direction for enterprise reform. Deng Xiaoping's veto of that suggestion signalled the end of workerist attempts to steer the reform agenda. After the elimination of conservative challenges to that agenda signified by the Fourteenth Party Congress in 1992, no significant barriers remained to the promotion of market values in academic or policy circles. Friedman was invited back in 1993, a significant gesture, given that his 1988 visit had been used to tarnish Zhao Ziyang, who was deposed and placed under house arrest after Tiananmen.

Spreading the word

That year also saw the establishment of the Unirule Institute in Beijing. Its founder, the English businessman Antony Fisher, had been converted to neo-liberalism after reading the *Reader's Digest* version of *The Road to Serfdom*. On Hayek's advice, Fisher took the think-tank route, founding the Institute of Economic Affairs in 1955, later a hot-house for Thatcherism. The Manhattan Institute followed, and in 1981, warming to his role as 'the Johnny Appleseed of the free-market movement', he founded the Atlas Economic Research Institute, later named the Atlas Network, which exists primarily for think-tank proliferation and

---

[40] Friedman's lectures and some of his conversations are published in Milton Friedman, *Friedman in China*, Hong Kong 2013.

funding.[41] The Unirule Institute was set up in 1993, as the Beijing affiliate of the Atlas Network.[42] While not the biggest economic think-tank in China, Unirule was the most ideologically focused, and over its twenty-five-year existence it sponsored conferences, symposia, seminars and other activities that drew participants from all levels of government, the media and the private sector.[43] Although it received no funding from the state, Unirule did consulting work and drafted research reports for a number of state agencies. Several of the most prominent economists associated with Unirule are also members of the Chinese Economists 50 Forum, established in 1998 in an effort to gather the country's most prominent and accomplished economists into one organization. Through the work of Unirule and its most active members, neo-liberal doctrine became part of the discourse in policy discussions at national and local levels. In establishing the criteria by which progress toward property rights, privatization, efficiency and increased competition could be measured, neo-liberal economists shaped policy, even though their specific recommendations often remained beyond the will of the state. The CCP leadership was more comfortable, officially, with economists along the neo-classical spectrum. Neo-liberal economists could, however, always point to the inadequacy of market measures so far undertaken, and thus serve as a goad for further reforms.

From Dale Carnegie to Steven Pinker, books on economics for popular audiences have contributed to the expansion of 'economic' epistemologies into nearly all aspects of life. Popularization of wisdom from the new discipline of economics, as reconstituted along market lines, took up that work in China as well. In the late 1980s and after, scores of economic texts from Adam Smith onwards were translated into Chinese. Von Mises and Hayek were hugely popular among general readers. At those bookstores that functioned as agenda-setting scenes for intellectual life—Xianfeng in Nanjing, Jifeng in Shanghai (now closed),

---

[41] John Blundell, 'The Life and Work of Sir Antony Fisher', Institute of Economic Affairs, 10 July 2013.
[42] The English name is a contraction of Universal Rule, or *tian ze* in Chinese. The classical source is a couplet from the poem 'Zheng min' in the pre-dynastic *Poetry Classic*: 'Heaven gave birth to our people, in form and in rules.'
[43] The Chinese Academy of Social Sciences sponsors work across the political spectrum. The China Center for Economic Research, established in 1994 by Justin Lin, is larger than the Unirule Institute, and arguably more influential.

Wansheng in Beijing—their work was featured prominently: at Jifeng right at the entrance. An early and comprehensive effort to introduce new economic thinking to a wider Chinese audience was the 14-volume *Shichang jingjixue puji congshu* [*Market Economics Popular Book Series*]. This had been initiated by the Chinese Economists Society, founded in 1985 by a group of US-trained Chinese economists working in the US and in China.[44] The series, deliberately written with a minimum of mathematical formulae, was aimed specifically at government officials, researchers, enterprise managers, and faculty and students in higher education, and was intended to provide this population with a broad basic knowledge of all areas of economics.

The first book in the series, *Mass Market Economics*, by Zhang Fan, was an introduction to micro-economics structured around the transition from a planned to a market economy, with comparisons between the two systems, in all cases to the detriment of the former. Volume Two was devoted to macroeconomic theory, and other volumes covered family economics, organizational structure and management, currency, securities markets, international trade and FDI. *The Visible Hand: The Role of the Government in Market Economies* and another volume devoted to public-choice theory (significantly, the only one concentrating on a particular school of economics) are explicitly ideological, as is the final volume in the series, and its biggest seller, *The Economics of Daily Life: Investigations into the US Market*. The latter was written by Mao Yushi, founding director of Unirule and China's most famous neo-liberal, based on his year as a visiting fellow at Harvard. A market-fundamentalist claim for the rationality and practicality of US economic life—topics range from home ownership to garbage collection and supermarkets—it concludes with that scenario beloved by neo-liberals, the prisoner's dilemma, and admonishes officials that:

> exchange has specific norms, based on human rights and market regula-
> tions. Respect for regulations cannot depend purely on self-interest. The
> prisoner's dilemma makes clear why market regulations are necessary,
> and why only an uncorrupt and efficient government can lead us toward a
> standardized market.[45]

---

[44] See the group's website at www.china-ces.org. The group also organized publication of a 12-volume *Modern Business Administration Book Series* in 1995.
[45] Mao Yushi, *Shenghuozhongde jingjixue*, Beijing 1993, pp. 252–7.

And contrary to the widespread suspicion of market transactions and motivations that characterized the early stage of the transition period, it argued for the morality of a well-run market economy.

Homo economicus sinensis

A growing body of work by Western scholars of neo-liberalism over the last ten years has described its social, political, subjective, epistemic and psychic dimensions. The latest, neo-liberal version of *homo economicus* is shaped by the extension of the economic and its attendant forms of measurement, evaluation and calculation to all aspects of life: by competition and risk as the primary modalities of existence; by a malleability of the self that comes from its fundamentally entrepreneurial nature; and by a vast reduction of the sphere of politics and political possibility. Epistemologically, it is free of transcendence or truth, the latter only realizable through the impersonal workings of the market. This version of the market requires government intervention and maintenance, but it is a situational and pragmatic version of governmentality, beholden to neither history, nor *telos*, nor first principles. The institutional supports for the construction of the neo-liberal subject are privatized and family-centred, with a diminution of collective or state-provided welfare guarantees. It is not only a polarized society, but is unapologetically— sadistically, some critics say—divided into winners and losers.[46]

With minor qualifications, this description applies to twenty-first century China, dating roughly from the 2001 accession to the WTO, when the consolidation of capitalism can be considered more or less complete.[47] Compared to its evolution in the West, the journey from the

---

[46] See among others Wendy Brown, *Undoing the Demos: Neoliberalism's Stealth Revolution*, New York 2015; Melinda Cooper, *Family Values: Between Neoliberalism and the New Social Conservatism*, New York 2017; Davies, *The Limits of Neoliberalism*; Pierre Dardot and Christian Laval, *The New Way of the World: On Neoliberal Society*, London and New York 2013; Byung-Chul Han, *Psychopolitics: Neoliberalism and New Technologies of Power*, London and New York 2017; Jamie Peck, *Constructions of Neoliberal Reason*, Oxford 2010. Foucault's lectures on biopolitics are important points of reference for these scholars: Michel Foucault, *The Birth of Biopolitics: Lectures at the Collège de France, 1978–79*, New York 2008.

[47] This periodization is Coase and Wang's view. It is also adopted by the editors of the online journal *Chuang* in their forthcoming 'Red Dust: The Capitalist Transition in China', probably the best account—from a communist perspective—of the emergence of capitalism in China: see www.chuangcn.org.

pre-reform political-economic order to a twenty-first century neo-liberal *homo economicus* was of far greater magnitude and speed. A precondition was the weakening of social and collective resources that would impede the consolidation of the isolated and entrepreneurial self and interfere with the operation of the market. This began in the 1970s with the dismantling of a democratic or participatory management culture in factories and workplaces, and the reduction of state or enterprise provision of child and family care, with women workers and retirees thereby required to take on most of the burden of social reproduction.[48] Workers' right to strike was eliminated in 1982. The older industrial working class employed in state-owned enterprises was decimated by lay-offs in the 1990s: by 1997 the elimination of 'iron rice bowl' lifetime (and inheritable) employment guarantees was virtually complete. De-collectivization of the rural sector, as even Coase and Wang complain, eliminated valuable organizational knowledge in agriculture. The privatization or closing of the Township Village Enterprises in the mid to late 1990s removed the last vestige of collective or cooperative ownership and management of factories. The new working class, comprising rural-urban migrants from peasant villages and laid-off workers in pre-reform industries, would face the labour market as isolated individuals, without social or organizational guarantees.

The rapid emergence of an 'ownership society' also contributed to the formation of the new subjectivity. There had been virtually no private housing in China prior to the late 1980s. The state began to encourage it in 1988, and through legal reform and other means facilitated home ownership through the 1990s. By 1998, when enterprises were forbidden to allocate housing to employees, there were over 24,000 real-estate firms in China, and the home-ownership rate was around 90 per cent, among the highest in the world. Home ownership quickly became a central ideological and cultural value. Men find it difficult to marry without owning somewhere to live, and home purchases remain the investment of choice for those with investment capital. As urban home prices skyrocket under the pressure of an investment economy with too few outlets for capital besides real estate, home ownership becomes another determinant of

---

[48] Joel Andreas, *Disenfranchised: The Rise and Fall of Industrial Citizenship in China*, forthcoming. Dong Yige, *From Textile Mill Town to iPhone City: Gender, Class and the Politics of Care in an Industrializing China (1949–present)*, PhD dissertation, Johns Hopkins, 2019.

society's winners and losers. Only in 2007, though, were property rights given reasonably full legal protection, and ownership remains more restricted than it is in much of the world. No property owner owns the land on which a dwelling is built, for example, and title to real property is for seventy years only. Although many expect the seventy-year title limit to be amended, these restrictions make ownership a political and ideological aspiration, in addition to being a cultural value: the vast majority of home-owners want a deepening and strengthening of property rights, and this of course adds to a politically conservatizing impulse. There is widespread popular opposition to a property tax, for example, due in large part to the perceived incompleteness of ownership.

China's audit culture, a feature of neo-liberal governmentality described by Davies and others, is pervasive, reaching from audits of Communist Party cadres themselves to all levels of educational institutions. In universities, the audit culture has become more and more demanding and consequential: departmental, divisional and university rankings determine budget allocations and salaries. The Chinese version of the Research Assessment Exercise is purely quantitative, with predictable effects on academic life. Pay-to-publish is pervasive, as is ghost-writing, plagiarism and the filing of a host of useless patents. The social-credit system, scheduled to be implemented by 2020, is probably best understood not as Orwellian surveillance, but as an extension of audit culture into individual economic and contractual life, more to do with the 'nudge' economy than with punitive state spying.

The entrepreneurial self and the psycho-economy of human capital formation are deeply embedded in the family, in institutions of audit culture such as schools and workplaces, in everyday consumption and in social media, including networking, dating and electronic gaming. *Fazhan*, or 'development', is commonly used for describing one's life trajectory. Since the 1990s, *chenggongxue*, or 'success-ology' has been a huge business, flourishing in expensive seminars, online courses and in the host of books that dominate urban and airport bookstores. Chen Anzhi is probably China's most prominent success-ologist, with book and video sales in the many tens of millions, beginning with his *Mai chanpin buru mai ziji* [*Sell Yourself, Not Products*, 2000]. He has written that the experience of seeing success guru Tony Robbins while a student in the US in the 1990s changed his life forever. Success-ology texts, Pun Ngai and Leslie Chang report, are probably the most popular books among women factory workers, many of whom dream of opening small businesses.[49]

The state also helps commodify the acquisition of human capital. In the late 1990s, it introduced the 'professional qualification certificate' (*zhengshu*) system, which by the 2010s offered certification for over a thousand professions—singer, marketer, psychotherapist and so on. A multi-billion dollar industry exists to prepare candidates for the qualification certificate examinations, mistakenly viewed by many as a sure path to employment in a given profession. Individuals commonly acquire multiple qualification certificates in order to keep options open and maximize employment possibilities. China's social-media 'influence economy', though it operates on Chinese platforms, provides myriad opportunities for self-marketing and self-fashioning. Besides the assiduous cultivation of online personae for social-status signification or dating, there are a host of remunerative online modalities. Gaming, as spectator sport, is quite lucrative. *Wanghong*, or internet celebrities, are highly paid, and influence marketing is a multi-billion dollar business in China, which has the largest e-commerce market in the world. Many aspire to *wanghong* status. The blurred division between buyer and seller makes everyone in the 'like' economy a real or potential influence marketer.

Contra

As the conventional wisdom has it, the 1980s witnessed the discovery of the self, the emergence of the individual out of late-Cultural Revolution authoritarian conformity. Most leftists in China today who were of age in the 1980s describe themselves as having been 'liberal' in those days, when the force of individualism had radical, anti-authoritarian possibilities. They became leftists in the early or mid-1990s, when the shape of the new dispensation grew clearer, when they realized that the individual had been prepared not for liberation, but for consumption and selfishness. For most on the left today, the pre-reform socialist past remains a key resource for resisting wholesale neo-liberalization. Although few leftists are deceived by the declared fealty of the CCP leadership to socialism

---

49 Pun Ngai, *Made in China: Women Factory Workers in a Global Workplace*, Durham, NC 2005; Leslie Chang, *Factory Girls: From Village to City in a Changing China*, New York 2009.

or Marxism, many nevertheless continue to believe in the Party's self-correcting capacity, and find spaces of possibility or forums for socialist advocacy in state initiatives. Thus we see leftist advocates for an expanded role for the state-owned enterprises, despite the fact that in structure, function and labour relations they are little different from private firms. There are left defenders of the One Belt, One Road initiative, who see in it echoes of Bandung, rather than a new version of imperialism.

Leftist academic intellectuals mostly support social movements, including those of workers, environmentalists and feminists, although restrictions on what they can publish, and their own desire to remain influential over government politics, inhibit them from offering overt support to movement activists. A particular feature of the social-movement scene in China is the relative absence of a theoretical or critical intellectual component. This closeness to the state has limited the appeal of academic leftism to younger generations. It is in the social movements that politically significant collectivities are formed, and these constitute the most meaningful alternatives to the hegemony of neo-liberal subjectivity. In workplaces, in rural villages, and among those sectors of youth growing discouraged about their prospects and dissatisfied with the kind of jobs, family life and consumption culture on offer, there is both the will and organizational capacity for collective action, albeit not always of long duration. That might change. But such efforts are ongoing largely without the influence of intellectuals.

Although leftist intellectuals are quick to criticize neo-liberals like Mao Yushi or Zhang Weiying, there is on the left very little critical work on neo-liberalism's penetration into the social fabric via the audit process, success-ology, the social-media economy and the myriad institutions, protocols and habits that constitute everyday neo-liberal culture.[50] Many leftist intellectuals are nationalists, and view China's singular emergence as an economic power beyond US control as a victory for a systemic alternative, or at least for the as-yet-unrealized possibility of one. That systemic alternative might be something like Wang Hui's 'anti-modernity modernization', referring to the long history of China's revolution, or Gan Yang's unity of the 'three traditions': Confucianism, Maoist revolution

---

[50] Much critical work is translated into Chinese, but I found it very surprising that although neo-liberal work—von Mises, Hayek, Friedman, Becker, et al—is widely translated and available, none of the texts cited in footnote 46 above have been translated. This may be in the process of being remedied. I hope so.

and Dengist reformism.[51] China's modernization is thus, necessarily, a distinctive modernization. Neo-liberalism, in this view, is largely a Western import, and can and should be resisted as such.

Like many neo-liberals, Coase didn't use the word 'neo-liberalism'. But the capitalism he celebrated in China, organically conforming to neo-liberal logic, was grown in Chinese soil, and it has taken deep roots. We will probably find out before long how well it weathers a serious crisis. In any case, recognizing it for what it is, a home-grown version of a globally dominant political-economic rationality—and Coase is useful here—will be an important part of forming a lasting and meaningful opposition to it.

---

[51] Gan Yang, *Tong san tong* (Uniting the Three Traditions), Beijing 2007.

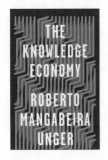

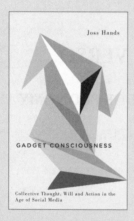

MONITQRED

BUSINESS AND
SURVEILLANCE
IN A TIME
OF BIG DATA

PETER BLOOM

PB 9780745338620
£16.99 | Jan 2019 | 272pp

Monitored:
Business and Surveillance
in a Time of Big Data

Peter Bloom

'The non-fiction equivalent of Orwell's *1984*. In a terrifying account of the new age of surveillance, Bloom demonstrates how Big Brother is actually Big Data'

SIMON SPRINGER, author of *The Discourse of Neoliberalism* and *The Anarchist Roots of Geography*

Gadget Consciousness:
Collective Thought, Will and
Action in the Age of Social
Media

Joss Hands

'Our obsession with gadgets is a key token of how deeply computer-based connection is now embedded in everyday life and consciousness. Joss Hands offers a highly thoughtful and theoretically astute reading of the possibilities for human reflexivity and agency that still remain'

NICK COULDRY, London School of Economics and Political Science

PB 9780745335346
£18.99 | Feb 2019 | 208pp

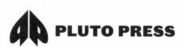

VICTOR SHIH

CHINA'S CREDIT CONUNDRUM

Interview by Robert Brenner

As a leading analyst of China's finance and economy, you were one of the first to identify and quantify the PRC's deepening debt problem and to warn about the implications of its slowdown. As background to this, could you give us your view of China's emergence as workshop of the world and second-largest economy on Earth? Clearly, its rise as the lowest-cost producer of a wide range of manufactures allowed it to secure, through imports, the increasingly complex capital goods and intermediate inputs required to climb the technological ladder, opening the way to an export-oriented growth path that was, at the same time, a particularly effective version of import-substituting industrialization (ISI). It also produced the enormous current-account surplus and huge reserves of foreign exchange, mainly in dollars, that meant China could effortlessly endow its non-financial corporations with the steady flow of loans and subsidies that underpinned their accelerated, investment-driven growth. But what made this possible? How did its initial rise come about?

CHINA'S EMERGENCE AS a major exporting power from the 1980s to the mid 2000s was ultimately founded on its rich endowment of cheap and relatively skilled labour, the freeing up of that labour force in the late 1970s by way of a de-collectivization that issued in an historic wave of agricultural commercialization and rural industrialization (Township–Village Enterprises, or TVEs), and the reduction of trade barriers in the advanced world, culminating in China's Most Favoured Nation (MFN) status and its joining the WTO at the start of the twenty-first century. The Soviet Union had

achieved a major industrial takeoff after World War Two in largely autar-
kic fashion, via ISI. China, by contrast, launched its industrial build-up
in the midst of the shift toward the globalization of the world economy,
in which it came to play the decisive role. Over time, as you say, China's
inexpensive labour—plus government subsidies and low-cost loans for
both domestic and foreign exporters—earned the country large trade
surpluses and sizeable foreign-exchange reserves. At their height the
latter totalled almost $4 trillion and provided China with the increased
bank deposits/money supply to finance the stepped-up lending that
underwrote the country's historic growth in GDP and investment.

*What role did China's integration into the already existing East Asian trade
and commodity chains play in this? It's often said that it was this network,
initially focused on Japan, Taiwan and Korea, that produced the capital goods
and intermediate inputs that were worked up into manufactured commodities
on the Mainland, and exported from there into the American market and the
other advanced-capitalist economies. Would you agree with that?*

Yes, I agree, but I would also highlight three further reasons why China
was able to take advantage of its central position in the emerging global
value chain so effectively. First, in terms of its size, and especially the
scale of its cheap labour force, China far surpassed Japan and the NICs
combined, with nearly a billion people even as early as the 1980s. This
huge population made for a continually growing labour supply, which
put downward pressure on labour costs, especially with the entry into
the labour market of perhaps 150 million migrant labourers from the
countryside. These workers were able to provide labour power at a particularly low price because they could subsidize their incomes from the
peasant plots that they never relinquished. Second, China's rise coin-
cided with major advances in information technology, which made
possible the construction of the sophisticated international communications and transportation networks through which the economy
expanded. Third, globalization and international free-trade agreements,
such as the WTO and NAFTA, brought substantial reductions in barriers
to imports throughout the world, opening the way for China to make
the most of its increasing cost advantages and competitive strength. The
PRC thus became part of the global production chain to a greater extent
than even Japan had managed. According to one study, China's imports

struck more industries in the US more quickly than any previous wave of imports.[1]

What about the role of the Chinese government in underwriting growth? How has China's organized capitalism, driven by subsidies and loans from state bodies at all levels—central, provincial, county, local—served to push growth forward?

What we have here is a kind of path dependence, where transnational producers across many light and increasingly also heavy industrial sectors came to rely on Chinese inputs for a growing part of their production chains. China has spent billions, even trillions, of US dollars on investments to maintain and expand its place in the global value chain. The support that its organized capitalism provides for this effort comes in part in the form of cheap land, world-class infrastructure, low taxes and cut-rate energy prices, as well as cheap credit for domestic exporters and, more and more, for firms competing with imported goods.

China's government, at all levels, has played an indispensable role in the provision of all these factors. Provincial, county and local administrations, much like state and city governments in the US, have been in competition with one another to attract investment to their localities, and they have done this by providing the greatest possible incentives to non-financial corporate producers and exporters—building infrastructure, developing land, offering credit, and so forth. In this way, they have enabled Chinese manufacturing to climb the technological ladder, producing increasingly complex goods, so as to be able to compete in an ever-broader range of manufacturing products.

You've said that China's vast export earnings and current-account reserves enabled it to grant large amounts of credit. What have been the implications for its currency?

There was a certain self-reinforcing logic to China's miraculous rise in the global production chain. That is, China's initial endowment of

---

[1] David Autor, David Dorn and Gordon Hanson, 'The China Syndrome: Local Labour Market Effects of Import Competition in the United States', *American Economic Review*, vol. 103, no. 6, October 2013.

cheap labour allowed it to generate those current-account surpluses by exporting—at least at first—light-manufacturing exports. Chinese exporters were paid by US and other overseas purchasers in dollars, or other national currencies, but exchanged them with their banks for yuan, because they needed the local currency to pay their Chinese workers, and to buy the capital goods and intermediate inputs that they secured domestically. The banks, in turn, would sooner or later exchange those dollars for yuan with the People's Bank of China (PBOC), the Chinese central bank, which added them to its dollar and other foreign-currency reserves. The result was, for an extended period, a swelling of renminbi deposits in Chinese banks, which could be lent on to non-financial corporations, and a spectacular ongoing rise of dollar reserves held by China.

All else equal, rising Chinese current-account surpluses and the corresponding build-up of dollar reserves would have meant the supply of dollars outrunning the demand for them. That would have put upward pressure on the value of the renminbi against the dollar, making for a process of renminbi revaluation that would have tended to undermine Chinese competitiveness, reducing its exports and its current-account surplus. But, committed as it was to export-led growth, the Chinese government adopted a series of measures to prevent the rise of the renminbi exchange rate that would otherwise have taken place.

Above all, it enforced a fixed, then minimally fluctuating, renminbi–dollar exchange rate. In order to accomplish this, it printed renminbi roughly to the extent necessary to cover the shortfall of demand for dollars vis-à-vis yuan that was the counterpart of the Chinese current-account surplus. It then used those yuan to purchase dollars on the international market, driving up what would otherwise have been insufficient demand for dollars to prevent the renminbi from rising and to sustain the exchange rate at a fixed level. This enabled China's current-account surplus to continue to rise while preventing the value of its currency from ascending along with it, maintaining China's competitiveness and sustaining its regime of export-led growth.

Without the PBOC's intervention, the build-up of dollars in Chinese hands could have not only led to an appreciating currency, but encouraged Chinese private investors to invest those dollars throughout the world, wherever they could secure the highest rate of return. But Beijing strictly limited the extent to which private investors could take money out of the country and deplete its foreign-exchange reserves by imposing a tight regime of capital controls. These controls have so far succeeded in preventing its emerging wealthy class from exporting too much capital, protecting China from the rampant capital flight seen in many developing economies, not to mention devastating runs on its currency.

China's dollar surpluses and reserves have thus remained largely in the hands of the central bank, rather than private investors. It has used them to further strengthen China's international position, by purchasing safe dollar-denominated US assets, specifically Treasury bonds and bills, as well as the debt of US government-sponsored entities, notably Freddy Mac and Fannie Mae. These huge purchases of US government debt brought about an enormous increase in the supply of credit to the US compared with the demand for loans, and thereby drove down the cost of borrowing in the US. The Chinese central bank has thus not only pushed up the value of the dollar, but driven down US interest rates. As a result, US consumers were able to borrow more easily and with a more valuable currency than otherwise. They have pushed up the demand for Chinese exports in relation to US imports, further increasing China's current-account surpluses and its dollar foreign-exchange reserves: a powerful virtuous circle underwriting Chinese expansion.

What were the implications of this for China's rise?

The beauty of this self-driving process was that it relieved China of the need to borrow from abroad to finance ISI, because it could rely for such financing on increases in the money supply. Money flowed into China in the form of dollars from current-account surpluses, foreign direct investment, and hot money inflows. The recipients of those dollars sold them to their banks in return for renminbi. The banks themselves secured the increased renminbi to cover the dollar deposits by exchanging the dollars with the PBOC. The PBOC purchased the increased inflow of dollars from the banks by printing high-powered money. So, indirectly, the creation of high-powered money—in the form of renminbi—by the PBOC allowed foreign-exchange earners to increase their renminbi deposits even while the exchange remained roughly at the same level.

At its height, in the mid 2000s, China's trade surplus rose to nearly 5 per cent of the money supply, significantly enhancing China's growth potential. The associated growth in the money supply, which continued at a rapid pace from the mid 1990s to 2008, was enormously significant. It allowed China to plough trillions of yuan in new credit to non-financial corporations to help maintain China's edge in global production, to climb up the technological value chain, and to pursue import substitution across an ever-larger range of goods, enabling the production and export from China of goods that formerly had to be purchased abroad.

This minimal dependence on external debt allowed China to pursue ISI without having to face the threat of a payments crisis, which so many other developing countries have had to confront—a crisis set off by the withdrawal of external debt that might be motivated by rising external deficits, collapsing currencies and capital flight. By the same token, China had little need to worry about speculation against the renminbi, because the massive inflow of dollars tended, all else equal, to drive up the renminbi rather than undermine it. China was thus able to employ an export-oriented path to industrialization to overcome the classical problem that had tended to confront, and sooner or later to disrupt, standard efforts at ISI in the postwar era. That problem was the tendency to incur uncontrollable current-account *deficits*, resulting from the growing cost of increasingly complex capital and intermediate imports to support the new domestic industries. By contrast, China's industrializers could solve this problem simply by virtue of their rising current-account surpluses.

Along with the rest of the world, in 2008–09, China entered the global economic and financial crisis. Its immediate result was the disruption of the markets for China's manufacturing exports, producing a sharp, and indeed permanent, reduction in the growth of demand for exports that had been driving Chinese GDP. The global economic crisis was a turning point for China, for it was at this moment that the country found itself obliged to begin to move away from the export-led model that it had followed for close to three decades, as its exports ceased to deliver the dollars that had enabled stepped-up lending. Could you explain what lay behind the crisis for China and how Beijing initially sought to deal with it?

In the wake of the global financial crisis, the growth of Chinese exports dropped precipitously, and the fact and form of the ensuing crisis suggested that China had reached a limit in achieving growth by way of exporting to the advanced-capitalist world. During the final years of China's boom, goods exports grew spectacularly, at around 20 per cent per year on average. But in 2009, Chinese exports plunged to minus 18 per cent. Export increases did come back fiercely, averaging 25 per cent per annum in 2010–11. By 2012, however, the honeymoon was over, and goods export growth collapsed to about 7 per cent per year for 2012–14, then *minus* 2 per cent for 2015–16. China's current-account surplus proceeded in a parallel manner. It had soared from 3–4 per cent of GDP in 2004 to 8–10 per cent of GDP in 2008–09. But it then dropped to 2 per cent of GDP in 2011 and continued at about the same level in the following years, through to 2016.

Even so, the constraint of collapsing exports did not materialize immediately, because the regime possessed ways to cushion the fall. The government's initial response to the fall-off in exports and ensuing economic downturn was to compensate for the plunge in demand from overseas by stoking demand at home. It turned to a Keynesianism of a familiar sort, but on an historically unprecedented scale. Wen Jiabao adopted a combination of an active fiscal policy and a loose monetary policy to implement a 4 trillion yuan ($580 billion) stimulus package for 2009 and 2010. Nevertheless, it was indicative of China's looming difficulties that a large portion of this pile of credit was channeled into stock and property markets rather than into the real economy—financial assets rather than capital goods and wages. As elsewhere, so in China, the gain in GDP for any given infusion of credit fell back significantly.

When the crisis hit in 2008–09, banks were so well capitalized and had so much liquidity that they could respond by boosting lending by over 30 per cent in the first year of the stimulus. Yet China could only follow this path forward for a limited period of time, because the current-account surpluses that had been accumulated during the export boom were used up rapidly by the historic stimulus programme, and the sharp decline in export growth prevented them from being replenished. The trade surplus and foreign-exchange flows ceased to infuse the banking system with the large new deposits which, in the past, allowed the banks to roll over illiquid assets comfortably while still financing new economic activities. China would have to find ways to infuse credit into the economy under much less favourable conditions.

How did the regime respond to the need to extend credit to drive growth, in the face of the diminution of the deposits that had long been provided by its towering current-account surpluses?

To maintain uninterrupted growth in the manner of its great boom, China would have had to generate a sizeable trade surplus, ideally in the region of 2–3 per cent of the money supply every year. But that would have required emerging markets in the developing world somehow taking over from the OECD economies, to provide China with increased export demand, larger current-account surpluses, increasing foreign-currency inflows and rising renminbi bank accounts—an impossible feat, as it turned out. China was therefore doomed to rely for increased lending on money creation by the People's Bank of China.

At their height in 2008, net foreign-exchange inflows over a 12-month period had made for an increase in bank deposits amounting to 7 per cent of bank assets. Even as late as mid 2011, net foreign-exchange inflows were still increasing deposits by the equivalent of 3.5 per cent of bank assets over a 12-month period. But 2012 was the end of the line. That year, foreign-exchange inflows were the equivalent of a mere 0.5 per cent of banks assets over a 12-month period. So, starting around 2012, in order to sustain growth, China began to expand credit simply by printing yuan, rather than relying on increasing renminbi bank deposits that derived from rising dollar inflows. Easy money creation from the foreign-exchange inflows had become a thing of the past.

Is this path to growth by way of creating ever greater debt, outrunning current-account surpluses, actually sustainable? What problems do you expect it to generate?

China faces an inherent contradiction between what it needs to do to maintain growth and keep its edge in the global production chain—which is to issue ever more credit—and what it needs to do to prevent the decline of the renminbi exchange rate and increasing pressure for capital to exit the country—which is to keep interest rates up and credit creation down. This contradiction has become more acute over time, because it's taking ever more credit to stimulate a given amount of growth.

In 2016, China needed three times as much credit to call forth the same amount of growth as in 2008. The scale of debt creation required to keep the economy moving forward has increased massively, and PBOC loans to domestic financial institutions rocketed from 4 trillion renminbi at the end of 2010 to 14 trillion renminbi by November 2017, a three-and-a-half-fold increase in the space of seven years. Total debt has grown from 163 per cent of GDP around 2009 to 328 per cent of GDP today, and this figure will likely continue to grow for the foreseeable future.

The bind that this extraordinary amount of debt creates for China is apparent in the huge levels of debt servicing—interest payments—it entails. In the twelve-month period ending in June 2017, the size of the *increase* in interest payments actually exceeded the increase in nominal GDP by 8 trillion renminbi. Since there were no large-scale defaults, the added interest burden must have been financed in some way. The increase in borrowing costs could, conceivably, have been paid for out of GDP (income) itself, directly reducing the growth of GDP. But, most likely, the new interest payments were covered by further loans, which made for a further rise in total debt. The Chinese economy has thus, by definition, become a Ponzi unit—engaging in what Hyman Minsky called Ponzi borrowing.

The upshot is that, if China wants to prevent the rate of growth from falling, it will have to continue to expand credit at a massive and ever-increasing rate, as it has been doing. But if the economy accumulates debt in this fashion, it will, unavoidably, drive down the value of the renminbi and create pressure for capital flight. Were the wall of capital controls to be substantially breached, it would open the way to financial crisis. If, on the other hand, China chooses to raise domestic interest rates so as to slow the growth of credit and shore up the currency, it will reduce the tendency for capital to leave the country but will also, at the same time, reduce the domestic lending and investment that has been so indispensable for sustaining growth.

It seems that China must choose between political stability—which requires growth and therefore a falling currency and rising debt—and financial stability, which means stemming capital flight and therefore a rising currency and slower growth of credit. The country seems to be coming up against the limits of its economic model. In the next three or four years, it will need to choose between, on the one hand, a large-scale devaluation resulting from the continuing build-up of debt, and, on the other hand, the bursting of the domestic financial bubble and an ensuing growth slowdown. It will be a tough choice that will test the Xi Jinping leadership.

In view of the contradictions inherent in depending on rising government-sponsored lending to drive growth, what policy responses are available to the Chinese regime?

The 2008–09 crisis and its sequels prompted several responses from the Chinese state. The smartest policy-makers in China understood the deepening contradictions and conflicts of interest built into the country's way of doing business. When Xi took office in 2012, he pushed for a slowdown in the expansion of debt, even though it would reduce the growth of GDP, under the slogan of the 'New Normal'. His advisers realized that the growth rate simply could not be sustained without putting enormous downward pressure on the renminbi, which would increase the pressure for capital flight and open the way to crisis.

The government therefore began to implement a series of steps to try to maintain stability as well as growth. First, slowing the pace of credit expansion—China has announced it is doing this, but whether it can actually accomplish it is not fully clear. Second, China needs to devote a larger share of what credit expansion does occur to fixed investment, to help it maintain its edge in manufacturing exports. It is therefore attempting to deflate asset-price bubbles, especially in land, real estate and equities, in order to reduce the incentive to engage in speculative as opposed to productive investment. Third, in the face of higher interest rates, China needs to secure more money to lend from what current-account surpluses and associated bank deposits and currency reserves it does accrue. The government is therefore committed to reducing banks' reserve requirements, at least to some extent. Finally, China needs to see what gains in trade it can secure by further developing the so-called Belt and Road Initiative—the network of ports, railroads and highways linking China to Europe across Central Asia and the Indian Ocean, on which the government is counting to further its commercial impact.

It is true that none of these policies has been fabulously successful, but in combination they have succeeded in stabilizing the level of the trade and current-account surplus as a share of the money supply. Without these policies, external surpluses would have shrunk to a negligible share of money supply by now. Still, the future looks at best uncertain. In the likely event that the growth of the US and European economies begins to slow in the coming year or two, China's trade and current-account surplus growth will also decelerate—and even with the recent effort to slow the increase of credit, in a slowing world economy, money-supply growth will outstrip that of the trade and current-account surplus. Sustaining debt-driven growth is going to become more difficult.

To what extent is the Xi Jinping government, with its 'New Normal' policy agenda, in sync with the Chinese elite, which prioritizes the consolidation and enhancement of its recently amassed wealth? Does this layer support the 'New Normal'?

The Chinese miracle has brought an astounding increase in economic inequality, with a polarization of wealth that has itself entailed an extraordinary concentration of riches in the top 1 per cent and above. In 2010–11, the wealthiest 1 per cent of urban households disposed of assets estimated at up to $5 trillion. Representing this new economic elite has naturally been a top priority for successive governments. Nevertheless, in attempting to do so, they have had to confront an array of difficult choices. Up to 2012–13 or thereabouts, declining real interest rates made for easy credit. But that entailed downward pressure on the renminbi, which meant a fall in the value of Chinese assets in international terms, and a corresponding drop off in the capacity to buy and invest abroad.

China's new rich, in possession of such a disproportionate share of the country's wealth, are not prepared to sit idly by and watch their assets being so brutally devalued. They have pressed, directly and indirectly, for a relaxation in the system of capital controls that has played such a central part in the country's growth strategy. They have not only tried to induce the government to slacken enforcement of capital controls, but have also attempted the sub-rosa export of capital themselves and sought to relocate their children to the US. The government, for its part, understands that capital controls constitute its ultimate line of defence in pursuing an independent economic strategy and has tried to protect that policy space even while avoiding controls that would be too draconian.

How has that been working?

Not too badly, at first. Until recently, the government managed to finesse the problem, because the banking system provided sufficient credit not just to nurture economic growth but to support various asset-price bubbles, from land to real estate to the stock market. The wealthy class was therefore able to make extraordinary profits by investing in China rather than abroad, by putting their money in markets for financial assets. Paradoxically, however, the 'New Normal' and the 'deleveraging' of the Chinese economy brought in by the Xi Jinping government began to short-circuit this form of money making, by deflating the various asset bubbles that had provided the wealthy elite with an alternative to capital flight.

As asset prices have fallen, the super rich have acquired a greater incentive to move their money out of the country, even though the government was hoping that slower credit growth would end up improving the long-term prospects for investment in China's real economy. Adding to the new turn to capital flight, the many risks associated with investing in China now included the political risk of getting pulled into a corruption scandal. If returns in China were no longer going to be extraordinary, Chinese investors might as well earn a more modest return in a much safer and more protected way overseas.

The 'New Normal' means in the first instance a slowdown in the growth of lending and of debt, for the sake of financial stability. But what about the longer run? What can the government do in qualitative terms to re-ignite China's economic dynamism?

In financial terms, the easiest thing to do is to copy what Japan did. In essence, the government can drive interest rates down to zero with massive quantitative easing, allow capital outflows and depreciate the currency, and issue a large quantity of government bonds to write down bad debt in the banking system. That could wipe out China's corporate debt almost overnight and make large-scale borrowing more sustainable, due to the near-zero interest rate. Were this to happen, exports would pick up, supported by a cheaper currency. However, for now, the leadership wants to avoid this approach, because growth would slow and the dollar value of China's economy would collapse, making it harder to catch up with the US economy in nominal terms.

To what extent does your analysis indicate that the export-based miracle is now behind us, due to the rise of manufacturing over-capacity in the world market and in China? Where does over-capacity fit into the story you have laid out?

Certainly, the combination of Chinese state control of the entire financial system and the lowering of trade barriers elsewhere allowed China to plough its trade surplus into massive investment in various industrial sectors and find demand in growing exports. If financial institutions had not been controlled by the government, private capital would have invested much more heavily overseas and in various services, from the beginning—diversifying its portfolio, so to speak, at the cost of manufacturing output and exports. However, due to the Chinese planners' priority on infrastructure construction and industrial capacity, the financial system devoted the bulk of its resources to these two areas, and this actually contributed to global over-capacity in a number of sectors, as China force-fed the build-up of fixed capital to aid the domestic production of goods that were already being made in the advanced capitalist countries, although at a higher cost.

In a sense one could say that China expanded through the systematic production of over-capacity in line after line, abroad and at home. This dynamic of over-supply generated trade shocks for industries and workers in advanced countries, as fixed investment soared and lower-cost Chinese goods squeezed the profits of producers abroad. But workers and corporations in China benefited mightily from it, as it detonated an unstoppable process of expansion that allowed China to avoid recession and unemployment for decades.

For China, the global crisis of 2008–09 was in the first instance a crisis of export markets: the upshot of China's way of appropriating market share via low-price, low-cost goods. Does it seem correct to understand this crisis of exports and the ensuing economic difficulties as an expression of a build-up of over-capacity originating in China and its credit-based wave of investment?

If we are talking about the domestic economy, I don't think, technically speaking, that over-capacity has been a major problem for China. This is because the regime can deal with the problem of demand in general—and problems of export demand in particular—simply by issuing more debt. Banks will, if necessary, roll over the distressed debt of money-losing state-owned enterprises (SOEs) and even of state-supported private firms. As we have said, this will lead to downward pressure on the currency, which could drive a crisis by way of capital flight. But this is why China has capital controls—precisely to prevent capital flight. So long as capital controls hold, this can go on forever.

But doesn't the reliance on credit to drive the economy in this way prevent the shakeout of low-profit businesses and means of production and so exacerbate over-capacity—further discouraging investment, to the extent that that depends on securing decent profits? Isn't the apparent rise in the amount of credit required to drive a given amount of economic growth evidence of this?

In the medium run, of course, over-capacity does cause a growing problem for policy-makers hoping to staunch capital outflows. There has been such a heavy focus on fixed capital investment in manufacturing industries for so long, with worsening over-capacity, that the rate of return has been driven low enough to discourage further investment. That has provoked a search for alternative investments outside industry, leading to a huge concentration on real estate, making for bubbles, as well as infrastructure. Should real estate and infrastructure also suffer a reduction in their rate of return, the pressure to invest overseas will soar and capital controls will be further tested.

Globally, this has caused major dislocations because banks in capitalist countries wouldn't support too many money-losing firms in sectors with over-capacity. Because intensive investment allowed China to build up its production capacity so rapidly, many firms in advanced countries, especially the United States, couldn't adapt—or could only adapt by moving production to China. Their creditors, unlike Chinese banks, wouldn't carry on providing credit to firms that could not compete with the 'China price', so thousands of firms either shuttered or relocated, leaving millions of workers unemployed, or employed in marginal jobs, in the space of less than a decade. Although much of the rhetoric about the incompatibility of capitalism and socialism reflects a Manichean construct of the Cold War, there are some deep incompatibilities between private capital and China's system of state-controlled capital.

Is China actually capitalist? It has that appearance to some degree, as it attracts investment for manufacturing exports on what would seem to be the capitalist criterion of a high rate of return—secured through relatively low wages and relatively high skills and technology. But what about the widespread refusal to allow firms to go out of business? What about the pressure from government bodies to have firms invest, no matter what their rate of profit? Where do capital controls fit in? How would you understand Chinese officialdom's access to income without directly investing in private enterprises?

Do the SOEs, like many state-owned firms elsewhere, adhere to capitalist norms and prioritize profit-making?

This is a tricky question to answer. I would still say that China has a system of 'state capitalism'—that is, although private households command trillions in financial and physical assets, the government still channels the vast majority of investment, both financial and in the real economy, into the areas it wants to support. The majority of assets held by Chinese banks, for example, are loans and bonds to finance state-sponsored projects or SOEs. Even Chinese households' love of property investment has been shaped by government policies to commodify land and housing, promulgated in the early 1990s—as well as by the lack of available alternatives, above all investing overseas.

You have repeatedly warned that there is a significant probability of a financial crisis in China, unless there is a big decline in the value of the renminbi. Could you unpack this for us?

As I have emphasized, the contradiction between the need to create credit, to drive growth, and the need to secure a stable currency, to avoid financial crisis, has intensified in recent years. In order to keep the economy turning over, the PBOC already had to carry out a devaluation in 2015, even if a relatively limited one. But this led almost immediately to major waves of capital flight in the fall of 2015 and in early 2016. This accounted for most of the trillion-dollar depletion of foreign-exchange reserves that took place over the period 2014–17, as wealthy citizens rushed their money out of the country. If the Federal Reserve were to increase interest rates in 2019, China would find itself in a still more precarious position. In a world where the interest rate on US treasury bonds, the safest assets in the world, rose to over 4 per cent, while Chinese bank deposits and government bonds offer a return of just 3.5 per cent, the temptation to move money out of China would be irresistible.

Prior to 2013, severe capital flight had been considered only a remote possibility in China. As late as the middle of 2014, foreign-exchange reserves still amounted to 20 per cent of the money supply. In subsequent years, however, the reduction of foreign-exchange reserves and the accompanying increase in the money supply cut the ratio between them to just 10 per cent. This meant that if households and firms were to move the equivalent of just 10 per cent of money supply out of the country, China's foreign-exchange reserves would basically be gone, leaving the economy profoundly vulnerable to a crisis triggered by capital flight, were the PBOC to continue to drive the economy by issuing more credit.

To stave off this eventuality, the Xi Jinping regime has implemented a series of radically escalating capital-control measures. These have included limits on corporations swapping renminbi into US dollars without underlying trade invoices, checks on the veracity of trade invoices to prevent over- and under-invoicing, higher hurdles for individuals to convert renminbi into dollars, and a crackdown on underground banks and popular offshore locations for currency exchange. These draconian steps have significantly restricted the exit of renminbi in the last few years.

But the fact remains that ongoing foreign trade still allows for the over- and under-invoicing of exports and imports, and the ability of Chinese citizens to take trips overseas means they can still whistle funds out of the country, with the consequence that a significant uptick in outflows of dollar reserves remains very possible. Indeed, if these processes were allowed to continue for long enough, they could easily lead to a crisis of confidence in the renminbi. The result might not be catastrophic, but a major devaluation implemented in response to capital flight would lead to several years of negative growth, some external default, and asset deflation. Were such a crisis of confidence in the currency to occur in lockstep with an international panic in the world's already highly vulnerable emerging markets, the squeeze on China could become very serious indeed.

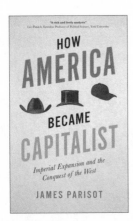

PB 9780745337876
£19.99 | Feb 2019 | 272pp

How America Became Capitalist: Imperial Expansion and the Conquest of the West

James Parisot

'There is a relatively limited literature covering the entire course of the USA's transition to a capitalist society. In his concise but illuminating new book, James Parisot provides such an account'

NEIL DAVIDSON, author of *How Revolutionary were the Bourgeois Revolutions?*

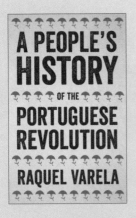

PB 9780745338576
£19.99 | Feb 2019 | 352pp

A People's History of the Portuguese Revolution

Raquel Varela
Edited by Peter Robinson
Translated by Sean Purdy

'Lively, brilliantly documented and filled with the voices of Portugal's ordinary people, this book recovers the revolution from below that shook Portugal in 1974-5'

COLIN BARKER, author of *Festival of the Oppressed: Solidarity, Reform and Revolution in Poland, 1980-81*

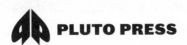

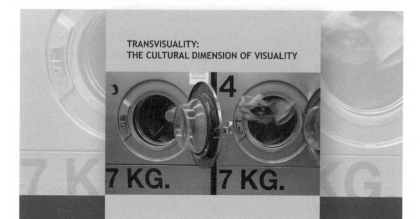

TRANSVISUALITY:
THE CULTURAL DIMENSION OF VISUALITY

VOLUME III: PURPOSIVE ACTION: DESIGN AND BRANDING
EDITED BY ANDERS MICHELSEN AND FRAUKE WIEGAND AND
CONTRIBUTIONS BY TORE KRISTENSEN

TRANSVISUALITY: THE CULTURAL DIMENSION OF VISUALITY (Volume 3)
Purposive Action: Design and Branding
ANDERSMICHELSEN, FRAUKE WIEG
AND TORE KRISTENSEN

In the contemporary and ever-changing society, 'the visual' has become a dynamic element of life which traverse all sort of different and diverse articulations – what is termed transvisuality. In this book such processes are researched from the particular vantage points of design of the visual and branding of the visual.

February 2018 • Hardback • ISBN 9781786941589

DIDIER FASSIN & ANNE-CLAIRE DEFOSSEZ

AN IMPROBABLE MOVEMENT?

Macron's France and the Rise of the Gilets Jaunes

O N 22 NOVEMBER, five days into the *gilets jaunes* protests, with some 2,000 roads and roundabouts barricaded across the country and 280,000 demonstrators having taken to the streets in the major cities, Emmanuel Macron welcomed journalists from *Le Monde* to the Élysée. It was not to give them his analysis of this extraordinary outburst but to take them on a tour of the presidential palace, where he had undertaken a costly renovation of its sumptuous ballroom. He told them that Brigitte, the First Lady, was supervising the project, and praised her choice of a €300,000 carpet woven at the Royal Manufactory of Aubusson. 'We are at a moment in the life of the nation when it is necessary to invest', he declared, and since the Élysée was the showcase of France, it had to be a priority.[1] For a president who regards the King's death during the Revolution as a permanent trauma for the French people, and considers it his mission to occupy the vacated space, this disconnect between the preoccupations of the nation and its head of state—the yellow vests were initially supported by 75 per cent of the population, according to opinion polls—could be called a Louis XVI moment, comparable to the Bourbon monarch's laconic diary entry for 14 July 1789, the day the Bastille fell: 'Nothing.'

The executive had simply not taken stock of the magnitude of the yellow-vest mobilization, nor of the accumulated grievances that lay behind it. The insurgency was regarded as one more episode of futile protest against its neoliberal reforms. The experience of Macron's first two years in office—the repeated failure of massive demonstrations to prevent his revisions of the labour code, overhaul of the state rail operator and cuts to pensions—led Paris to believe that it could ride out this latest unrest. It deemed trivial the yellow vests' main complaint: an increase in fuel tax of 6.5 cents per litre for diesel and 2.9 cents for petrol, scheduled for 1 January 2019 and coming on top of similar rises implemented in 2018. The stated purpose of the carbon tax was to reduce fossil-fuel consumption, an ecological gesture intended to dispel the negative impression created by the resignation of Nicolas Hulot, the popular environment minister, who had declared himself frustrated by the government's lack of political will on green issues.

Persuaded of their strength and of the weakness of the mobilization against them, the President and his ministers initially refused to listen to the demonstrators. Macron instead tried to discredit them as 'a heinous mob' and latter-day 'Poujadists'—a reference to the populist anti-tax campaigners of the 1950s, whose discourse had included anti-intellectual, xenophobic and antisemitic themes. The spokespersons for the *gilets jaunes* 'target Jews, foreigners, homosexuals', he alleged, even though the movement had, since its inception, rejected all self-proclaimed representatives.[2] Christophe Castaner, the interior minister, labelled the activists 'seditious far-rightists'—despite their adamant refusal to associate with any political party—and compared them to the Taliban for the (possibly accidental) destruction of a garish sculpture on a roundabout in Châtellerault on 16 December, after a barricade was set on fire to forestall an attempt by police to clear the road.[3]

Truth be told, very few politicians or commentators had anticipated such disturbances, or proved able to interpret them once they became entrenched—despite a burgeoning literature on the subject. How could a leaderless grassroots movement, involving often quite small groups of protesters, monopolize the national news, capture the attention of the wider world and destabilize a government that had swept to power by a landslide victory in 2017? As Jacques Rancière has suggested, it is as difficult to understand why some people mobilize when confronted with situations they regard as unacceptable, as it is to understand why others

---

[1] Louis Nadau, 'Pendant ce temps-là, Emmanuel et Brigitte Macron reçoivent *Le Monde* . . . pour parler déco de l'Élysée', *Marianne*, 5 December 2018.
[2] Emmanuel Macron, 'Mes vœux 2019 aux Français', 31 December 2018.
[3] 'Gilets jaunes: Castaner compare l'incendie d'une statue à la destruction des Bouddhas par les talibans', LCI, 18 December 2018.

in similar or even worse circumstances do not.[4] The *gilets jaunes* upsurge appears all the more remarkable when one considers that most of its adherents had never participated in a demonstration before and refuse any political or union affiliation. One should therefore be prudent when interpreting an event that has either been described as a phenomenon without precedent or likened to movements as varied as the revolutionary *sans-culottes* and Italy's Cinque Stelle.

Condescensions

Commentators who derided the initial grievance of the *gilets jaunes* ignored the fact that opposition to the fuel-tax increase had a deeper meaning, rooted in the social transformations of the past decades, which recent measures have merely aggravated.[5] Worsening economic inequality since the 1980s was relatively well tolerated as long as living standards continued to improve for everyone, even if not at the same pace. But since the 2008 financial crisis, the income of the bottom 40 per cent of the population has dropped. Pauperization has mainly afflicted those who were already the most disadvantaged, among whom joblessness and under-employment became increasingly rife. At the same time, the cost of housing, energy, insurance and school meals has risen faster than the overall rate of inflation. These trends have left the lowest segment of the population with a reduced budget to meet all their other needs.

In parallel, rising rents and house prices, especially in large cities, have forced more and more people on tight incomes to move further away from urban centres, where many of them work. Public transport remains chronically underdeveloped in these hinterlands, so owning a car is essential. The soaring cost of fuel has therefore eaten into household budgets. In rural areas the problem is even more acute. There, the atrophy of public services—from post offices to train stations, hospitals to schools—obliges people to drive into larger towns to access any sort of amenity. Thus, whereas the tax increases had little impact on privileged social layers, since fuel represents only a small proportion of their budgets, they constituted a real financial burden for people living at a distance from the cities. It is estimated that the carbon

---

[4] Jacques Rancière, 'Les vertus de l'inexplicable—à propos des "gilets jaunes"', AOC, 8 January 2019.
[5] Xavier Molénat, Guillaume Duval and Vincent Grimault, 'Inégalités: Les cinq fractures françaises', *Alternatives économiques*, 21 December 2018.

tax weighs five times more heavily on the bottom decile than on the top, even though the former produces much less pollution than the latter. Besides, the car industry itself was exempted from this environmental levy. On top of these injustices, drivers of diesel cars saw the extra tax hike for their vehicles as being particularly unfair, because the government has encouraged the use of this type of engine for decades, and so it is found today in more than 60 per cent of all personal vehicles in France—mostly the older ones owned by lower-income road-users. Mocked as archetypal rednecks by government spokesperson Benjamin Griveaux, the 'drivers of diesel cars who smoke fags' thus had every reason to don a yellow tabard.[6] It is obvious that the Parisian commentariat, which enjoys the use of chauffeurs, Uber and the Métro to move around the city, as well as hybrid cars stowed away in the country houses where they spend their weekends, has had a difficult time understanding these earthly concerns about a several-cent increase in the price of fuel.

This contemptuous attitude, fully shared and overtly expressed by the authorities, who see the protesters as 'stupid, brutal, thugs, fascist, reactionary, vulgar'—in the words of David Guilbaud, a high state official, quoting the language of his colleagues—has reinforced the sense of social relegation among the disregarded classes.[7] The President himself has made multiple disparaging or condescending public interventions of this kind: dismissing his critics as 'slackers and cynics'; describing women laid off from a slaughterhouse as 'mostly illiterates'; drawing a contrast between 'people who succeed and people who are nothing'; deploring that 'we are putting crazy amounts of dough into minimum social benefits'; telling a young jobseeker that 'I'll cross the street and I'll find you something'; and commenting, in reference to the yellow vests, that 'we must make those who suffer hardship take responsibility because some behave well but others screw around'.[8] These incendiary statements, which a late act of contrition in his television address of 10 December could not erase from collective memory, probably explain why the January polls showed that 68 per cent of the French population find Macron arrogant and that he is the most unpopular French president in

---

[6] Jean-Michel Bretonnier, 'Environnement: Cette France qui roule au diesel et fume des clopes', *La Voix du Nord*, 30 October 2018.

[7] David Guilbaud, '"Égoïstes, imbéciles, illuminés, poujadistes, vulgaires": les Gilets Jaunes vus depuis une certaine haute fonction publique', AOC, 19 December 2018.

[8] Cyril Brioulet, 'Maladresse ou arrogance: les dix phrases choc d'Emmanuel Macron', *La Dépêche*, 17 September 2018.

the history of the Fifth Republic, with only 23 per cent holding a positive opinion of him.[9] As the historian Gérard Noiriel notes, 'popular struggles almost always involve the denunciation of the disdain of the powerful, and that of the yellow vests only confirms this rule.'[10]

But Macron's verbal haughtiness is not the only cause of the spectacular collapse in his approval ratings. For the protesters, his deeds, more than his words, manifest his scornful indifference to their condition. The first actions of the newly elected President left no doubt about his political orientation. To the applause of business leaders, the former Rothschild banker abolished the solidarity tax on wealth, replacing it with a levy on real estate from which financial assets were exempt, and cut corporation tax as well as employer payroll charges. Conversely, to balance the state's budget, housing benefit, family allowances and pensions were all reduced. Not surprisingly, Macron soon earned the sobriquet 'President of the rich'. His justification for these policies rested on the hackneyed trickle-down theory, according to which reduced taxes on the wealthy and corporations stimulate investment, create jobs and eventually prove beneficial to all. But this did not convince the majority of the population, who understood that the man they had elected because he claimed to be neither right nor left was in fact a typical neoliberal. Far from rejuvenating the political world, as he had promised during his campaign, Macron seemed merely to represent the old politics in new garb.[11] This is probably why the yellow vests immediately obtained such an extraordinary measure of public support, despite the disruption they are causing to many people's daily lives. Although the number of protesters on the streets on any given day has rarely exceeded 100,000, the majority of the population who expressed sympathy with them in the polls should be regarded as demonstrators by proxy.

Unidentified political object

But is it even legitimate to call the protests of the yellow vests a movement? Several features of those protests run against this characterization, particularly if one considers how the mobilization developed in the closing weeks of 2018. First, rather than being a coordinated demonstration,

---

[9] Ipsos Public Affairs, 'Le baromètre de l'action politique', 16 January 2019.
[10] Gérard Noiriel, 'Les "gilets jaunes" replacent la question sociale au centre du jeu politique', *Le Monde*, 27 November 2018.
[11] Didier Fassin, 'Sure looks a lot like conservatism', *London Review of Books*, 5 July 2018.

it is a spontaneous uprising. Blockades are agreed upon between neigh-
bours and friends. Improvised protests take place at venues chosen at
the last minute via social media. Most of the time, no permission is
solicited from the authorities, which have been all too ready to declare
these rallies illegal and proceed to make arrests among anyone gathered
in a group. Second, no leaders or spokespersons emerged from their
ranks. Those who put themselves forward to liaise with the authorities
or accepted invitations onto talk shows were immediately criticized, and
sometimes even threatened. Third, no single watchword or programme
unified the participants. Although certain themes recurred, on tax justice in particular, the most frequent slogans heard were against Macron
himself, confirming the general mood of disaffection with the President.
This unconventional mobilization can be regarded, at least in part, as a
consequence of Macron's strategy of marginalizing 'intermediate bodies': traditional parties, crushed at the polls, with the exception of the
National Front; trade unions, discarded in the labour-reform process;
and non-governmental organizations, which the President has simply ignored. In conformity with his lofty conception of the sovereign,
Macron wanted to have 'the people' as his only interlocutor. Upon discovering that his honeymoon with voters had ended, however, with only
28 per cent of the population declaring they trusted the President—the
lowest-ever score in the annual poll on institutions—he was discounte-
nanced and paralyzed.[12]

Opposition parties and the unions were also disconcerted by this pecu-
liar mobilization, with its obscure social base, unusual practices and
unclear aims—all the more so since it somewhat discredited their
own, less effective forms of action to contest the government's policies. Politicians were hesitant to support a protest wave depicted by the
authorities and the mainstream media as violent, uncontrollable and
leaning to the far right. They were all the less inclined to do so since the
protesters strongly rejected all attempts to instrumentalize their struggle. It was Jean-Luc Mélenchon's Les Insoumis who most openly backed
the yellow vests, while Marine Le Pen's Rassemblement National did so
in a more discreet and perhaps more effective way. Polling about voting intentions for the May 2019 elections to the European Parliament
indicates that the latter has benefitted more from the crisis than the former, whose constituency has dropped. Meanwhile the core of Macron's

---

[12] Madani Cheurfa and Flora Chanvril, '2009–19: la crise de la confiance politique',
Baromètre de la confiance politique, SciencesPo Cevipof, January 2019.

support remains solid.[13] For their part, the major unions stated that they understood the anger of the yellow vests and shared their concern about purchasing power, although they were more cautious when it came to the demand for reduced taxation, since tax is the main instrument for redistribution. Locally, however, in Marseilles for instance, trade unionists joined the protesters, arguing that they shared much in common.

A major reason for the discomfort felt by public figures is the difficulty of apprehending who the protesters are. It is certainly the case that the very form taken by the mobilization renders any analysis of its socio-demographic composition problematic. However, studies have been done *in situ* at the roundabouts, via social media and through opinion polls.[14] The observations gleaned so far by journalists and sociologists across the country do suggest some general traits. First, the yellow vests are a very heterogeneous group. Most have no experience of engagement in social movements, organized labour or political parties. Second, they combine men and women—the latter unusually well represented, at 45 per cent of the total—pensioners and workers, craftsmen and tradesmen, nurses and housekeepers, students and unemployed. Most adherents come from the upper-working class or the lower-middle class, drawn together by the shared experience of their income being progressively squeezed by tax hikes and rising expenses. Third, most reside in the distant outskirts of cities, as well as in depopulated rural areas, where there is a painful sense of abandonment by the state. The expression 'peripheral France', so often used to characterize them, should thus be taken in the polysemous sense of those who occupy—or regard themselves as occupying—a political, social and spatial periphery. In the opinion of sociologist Serge Paugam, the yellow-vest movement represents 'the revenge of the invisible' against the 'social contempt' of the elites.[15]

But as the geographer Hervé Le Bras has shown, contrary to a common perception, the movement's distribution across the country does not run in parallel to the far-right vote. Nor does it cluster in the most

---

[13] Ifop, 'L'intention de vote à l'élection européenne de mai 2019', 16 January 2019.
[14] Benoît Coquard and Eric Aeschimann, 'Des femmes, des abstentionnistes, des bandes de copains ... Un sociologue raconte les gilets jaunes', *BibliObs*, 1 December 2018; Collectif, 'Qui sont vraiment les "gilets jaunes"? Les résultats d'une étude sociologique', *Le Monde*, 26 January 2019; Luc Rouban, 'Les "gilets jaunes", une transition populiste de droite', *The Conversation*, 28 January 2019.
[15] Serge Paugam, 'Face au mépris social, la revanche des invisibles', *AOC*, 7 December 2018.

impoverished territories.[16] Significantly, Seine-Saint-Denis, which is the most deprived French department, with a large immigrant population, has seen neither road blockades nor street demonstrations. This is indeed, paradoxically, one of the most obvious and yet least noticed characteristics of the *gilets jaunes*: they do not include the most disadvantaged social elements of all. The denizens of housing projects administratively named 'neighbourhoods in difficulty' or 'urban sensitive zones', where socioeconomic and ethnoracial segregation is most pronounced, have been absent from the mobilization, in contrast to their leading role in previous bouts of unrest. Mostly of African descent, they suffer the highest rates of unemployment and poverty. Many households do not own a car. They see very little investment in public services, encountering the state in the form of law-enforcement officers rather than social workers. Their schools are chronically short of teachers. When interviewed, they declare that they do not really identify with a movement that is mostly white. While not expressing disapproval of the protests, they nevertheless find it ironic that the yellow vests seem to be discovering what they have experienced themselves for decades: social marginalization, economic hardship and police violence—processes no one seemed to care about until now.[17]

Popular power

Although the revolt has articulated an extraordinarily diverse range of grievances, there are two major themes running through the yellow vests' programme: social justice and democratic renewal.[18] The first of these themes is principally focused on taxation, with recent changes in the tax code deemed wholly unfair. The most popular demand is for the restoration of the solidarity tax on the wealthy. But the issue of purchasing power is also central. This translates into a call for increases to the minimum wage and minimum pension. Interestingly, the discourse of the yellow vests displaces the social question from the traditional focus on poverty to a more explosive discussion about inequality. For instance, they propose a more progressive tax system, the abolition of lifelong

[16] Pascal Riché, 'La carte des "gilets jaunes" n'est pas celle que vous croyez', *L'Obs*, 21 November 2018.
[17] Éric Marliere, 'Les "gilets jaunes", vus par les quartiers populaires', *Slate*, 9 January 2019.
[18] Jérémie Chayet, 'Liste des 42 revendications des gilets jaunes', *Mediapart*, 2 December 2018.

benefits for former presidents, and a maximum of twenty-five students per class to help improve the very poor performance of France's education system in comparison with other countries. They also express their solidarity towards the most disadvantaged. Among the forty-two demands that the protesters eventually compiled in January, one was for 'zero homelessness'—one of Macron's promises before his election—and another was for better treatment of asylum-seekers, including improved security, housing, food and education. Contrary to the French President's insinuations, and confounding the hopes of Matteo Salvini, Italy's interior minister, who pledged the yellow vests his support, the majority of protesters did not manifest any hostility toward migrants. Instead, they called for 'a real politics of integration'. This positioning does not, of course, preclude a sympathy for the far right among a minority of participants.

On the other hand, the shortcomings of France's representative democracy were unreservedly denounced. With a president chosen by less than 25 per cent of the electorate in the first round of voting, and a parliament lacking a single blue-collar representative—20 per cent of the active population—neither the executive nor the legislative branch can be said to properly represent the people. Moreover, the presidentialist cast of the Fifth Republic has taken an extreme form in the past two years, as Macron implements his 'Jupiterian style', bypassing parliament to decide on everything himself, dismissing all mediations.[19] Opposing this autocratic form of governance, in which the sovereign only thinks of his relation to the people in pedagogical terms—to explain to them why he governs the way he does—the yellow vests propose acephalous assemblies, egalitarian debates and solidarity practices. Their flagship proposal is for the consultation of the population by referendum, on topics petitioned by the citizenry, without the intervention of either president or parliament, as is the practice in Switzerland and Italy. They also demand an extension of the president's term of office from five to seven years, so that representatives are no longer elected immediately after the head of state, which virtually guarantees that the majority of the National Assembly will belong to his party and docilely follow his instructions. For the *gilets jaunes*, such a constitutional change would help to make

---

[19] Hélène Combis, '"Président jupitérien": comment Macron comptait régner sur l'Olympe (avant les Gilets jaunes)', *France Culture*, 11 December 2018.

'the people's voice heard'. Of course, many on the left have long been much more radical, pressing for a Sixth Republic.

The heterogeneity of the yellow vests, the diversity of their demands and, more than anything, their success with public opinion, has led to erratic and contradictory reactions on the part of the government. Three moments in particular stand out. Initially, while the President remained silent for an unusually long period of time, his government held fast to its policies, expecting that the mobilization would peter out as the Christmas holiday approached. Prime Minister Édouard Philippe declared that the minimum wage would not be raised, since this would be inconsistent with the reduction of levies on corporations, and that the tax increase on fuel would be maintained in the name of environmental protection. In the supposed contest between those who worry about what they have left at the 'end of the month' and those more concerned about the 'end of the world', the government was on the side of the latter—a rhetorical position that rings hollow, given Macron's regressive policies on pesticides, nuclear plants and the extractive industries.

Then, as the protests continued and some politicians within the presidential majority called for a less dismissive attitude, a series of concessions were made, with ambiguous implications for social inequality and economic stability. The fuel increase was postponed and eventually cancelled altogether. The minimum wage was raised via a special premium paid by the state instead of the employer, thus transferring the cost to taxpayers. Overtime payments were stripped of taxes and charges—irrelevant for employees at the bottom of the pay scale, who do not make enough money to pay tax on their earnings. Retirees on the lowest income received an exemption from a new surcharge, yet pensions were de-indexed from inflation for the first time, making it possible for their real value to decline. Basic welfare benefits were not raised, and the solidarity tax on wealth was not restored. This package of measures was presented by Macron as a major 'social turn', but it did nothing to help the most precarious segments of the population, while sparing the corporate world and the most privileged, and also placed a heavy burden on the state's finances, deepening its deficit and auguring further cuts to public services.

Finally, on 13 January, confronted with continuing unrest, the President attempted to circumvent the yellow vests and arrest their momentum by announcing a 'great national debate', lasting three months and open to everyone. Although this was presented as a shift from the vertical style that has characterized Macron's first years in power to a more horizontalist mode of governing, there are many indications that the President has rigged the whole process. The four themes and eighty-two questions to guide the discussion were all decided in advance.[20] They correspond in part to reforms that were already in preparation—for instance, the reduction of the number of representatives and senators—and use formulations that predetermine the response: 'To decrease taxes and reduce the debt, which public expenditures must be cut in order of priority?' Certain topics deemed crucial by the yellow vests—citizen referenda, restoration of the solidarity tax on wealth, measures to increase people's purchasing power—have been excluded *a priori*. Others have been added despite bearing no relation whatever to the protesters' demands, sometimes with a clearly divisive intention. This is particularly the case with the questions on *laïcité*, which merely perpetuate the state's targeting of France's Muslim minority—'How do you propose to strengthen secularist principles in relations between the state and the religions in our country?'—and immigration, which pander to the conservative party, Les Républicains: 'Do you wish us to establish annual quotas defined by parliament?' The organization of the debate is under the control of two ministers, and the framework for analysing the information produced is opaque. The National Commission for Public Debates, which had been asked to oversee the process so as to ensure its transparency and neutrality, decided to withdraw, as its proposals had not been respected. The Commission's president, Chantal Jouanno, criticized the debate's lack of impartiality and its paternalistic orientation. In an opinion poll on 21 January, the majority of people had a positive view of the initiative, but 62 per cent thought that the government would not take what came out of it into account. Among people sympathetic to the yellow vests, this pessimism was even more widespread—79 per cent.[21]

State of repression

While the triangulations of Macron and Édouard Philippe may have shifted over time, one element has remained constant since the unrest

---

[20] Lucas Mediavilla, 'Grand Débat: les 82 questions soumises aux Français sur Internet', *Les Échos*, 16 January 2019.
[21] OpinionWay, 'Pour 67% des Français, le Grand débat national est "une bonne chose"', LCI, 22 January 2019.

began: the exceptional harshness of the repressive measures taken against the protesters. According to the criminologist Fabien Jobard, the number of persons injured 'exceeds everything that has been seen in France since May 1968'.[22] More people have been wounded by police weapons in two months than in the previous ten years. In the absence of data from the interior minister, a non-exhaustive count of casualties by the Against State Violence collective, confirmed by independent journalist David Dufresne, indicates that 111 individuals had been seriously wounded by the first week of January.[23] Most injuries were caused by Flash-Ball rubber-pellet guns and Sting-Ball grenades, riot-control devices that are not used in most European countries. An eighty-year-old woman died after being hit by a grenade. Three individuals fell into a coma after they were shot with a rubber ball. Four had a hand blown off. Eighteen lost an eye. Two-thirds of the victims were shot in the head, causing brain injuries, even though the weapons in question are supposed to be targeted at the trunk and limbs. A war reporter, who had avoided injury while covering Bosnia, Afghanistan, Libya, Chad, Iraq and Syria, was wounded for the first time in Paris. Indeed, people filming the demonstrations, including journalists, were specifically targeted by the police.

On 15 January, Christophe Castaner declared that he 'was not aware of any policeman or gendarme who had attacked yellow vests'.[24] His denial signalled that the government would support law-enforcement agents, whatever degree of physical force they resorted to. Five days later, confronted by critics about what they called 'state lying', a government spokesperson finally acknowledged the existence of 81 investigations conducted by the Inspectorate of the National Police into violence perpetrated by officers. However, the unusual brutality of the police cannot simply be attributed to the initiative of rank-and-file agents; it is the consequence of the recent evolution of state policies. After the terrorist attacks of 2015, a state of emergency was declared. Two days before it officially ended on 1 November 2017, Macron put a new security law to a vote in parliament.[25] It included most of the measures until then limited

[22] Fabien Jobard, 'Face aux "gilets jaunes", l'action répressive est d'une ampleur considérable', Le Monde, 20 December 2018.

[23] Désarmons-les, 'Recensement provisoire des blessé-es des manifestations du mois de novembre-décembre 2018', 4 January 2019.

[24] Anthony Berthelier, 'Ces gilets jaunes furieux de la petite phrase de Castaner sur les violences policières', HuffPost, 15 January 2019.

[25] Paul Cassia, 'Sortie de l'état d'urgence temporaire, entrée dans l'état d'urgence permanent', Mediapart, 31 October 2017.

to the state of emergency, in particular the extension of the prerogatives of the police and the licence to prohibit demonstrations. Powers originally justified as necessary for anti-terror operations have become the habitual form of police intervention to control protests. This includes the presence of snipers on the roofs of buildings—confirmed by police unions—the possession of assault rifles and the use of mutilating weapons. What was the exception has become the norm.

Spectacle of violence

Remarkably, however, during the first six weeks of protests, the national and international media remained completely silent regarding these casualties. They did not report on the violence of the police; they were instead mesmerized by the violence of the crowd. Television broadcasts played images of destruction and looting on the Champs-Élysées over and over again. Newspaper front pages showed night photos of barricades on fire, while editorials described scenes of chaos. During the demonstration of 5 January, a former boxing champion was filmed punching a police officer, who protected himself behind his shield and was only slightly injured. This made the headlines for several days, generating indignant reactions from the government, police unions and media pundits. No mention was made of the seven individuals who, that same day, had been seriously wounded by police, suffering brain injuries, facial wounds or the loss of an eye. The reasons why most media outlets produced this selective representation of the movement are probably multiple: they relied excessively on the official version of events put out by the authorities; some anticipated the expectations of their proprietors, who are often connected to the government, while others simply felt contempt toward the yellow vests; above all, they looked for stories and images that would attract an audience.

As the sociologist Laurent Mucchielli has written, 'violence produces effects of astonishment/fascination/repulsion which prevent thinking'.[26] In that regard, sensationalist footage and alarmist accounts may lead the public to forget that the presence of violent groups or individuals has been a common feature of French protests for decades and that, in the case of peasant unrest, public edifices were burned down, without provoking such an outcry. The violence at some *gilets jaunes* rallies is

---

[26] Laurent Mucchielli, 'Comment analyser sociologiquement la colère des Gilets Jaunes?', *Mediapart*, 4 December 2018.

undisputable. However, the defacement of the Arc de Triomphe during the 1 December protest in Paris inspired more emotion and denunciation than the deaths of eight people killed by the collapse of a dilapidated building in the centre of Marseilles, where local residents and yellow vests demonstrated peacefully on 2 December against the appalling housing conditions of the poor—as if the 'violence' of graffiti on a national monument was more scandalous than the violence of lethal negligence by public authorities. And when Macron claimed accusingly that ten people had died because of road blockades, he was actually referring to the unfortunate victims of traffic accidents caused by vehicles trying to go through or around the barricades.

By focusing exclusively on the violence of a minority of protesters, and of the rioters who infiltrated their ranks, while ignoring the brutality of the police, the media has dutifully contributed to the official narrative of events and to the normalization of the violent policing of protests. On 5 December, for instance, the government declared that the protesters were ready to descend on the capital 'to destroy and kill'. One frustrated *gilet jaune* resorted to addressing a television broadcast on Facebook: 'thousands of peaceable yellow vests near the Opéra, in Paris—will you show these images?' Responding to the pro-government slant of most media outlets, and their biased representations of the protests, the yellow vests have often showed hostility towards journalists, sometimes even assaulting them, and prefer to rely instead on social media and alternative news sites, where useful information as well as fake news abounds.

The irony is that the very mediasphere that has rightly been accused of vilifying the yellow vests and misrepresenting their protests has also given their movement the oxygen of publicity. Without the extensive coverage that they have enjoyed from the start, it is very unlikely that they would have received such extraordinary public attention. After all, other mobilizations in recent years have brought people out onto the streets without eliciting much interest, and a protest against a tax increase on fuel was not, on the face of it, a very exciting topic. What made a difference in the case of the yellow vests was the spectacle of violence. This is another paradox to be emphasized. The very images and narratives that showed the protesters in a negative light made them an attraction worldwide. This was not mere chance. Symbolic places and monuments were deliberately chosen as the stage for the crowd's performance. Because the destructions and lootings during the third demonstration on 1 December mostly took place in France's famed capital, the protest became a global phenomenon, eliciting supportive comments from across the political spectrum, from Salvini on the right to Sahra Wagenknecht on the left. It also generated similar mobilizations, from Belgium to Taiwan, and in Egypt a lawyer was sent to prison for having posted a picture of himself wearing a yellow vest. The French government now had to take this seriously. The majority of the population, although disapproving of the excesses of the crowd, continued to sympathize with the mobilization, as if it considered the physical violence of the protesters a comprehensible—if not justifiable—response to the structural violence of society.

Sense and uncertainty

So close to the start of the yellow-vest mobilization, it is difficult to draw definitive conclusions about its meaning and future. The movement has too often been treated as *sui generis*, when in fact useful comparisons can be drawn with mobilizations that have occurred in Spain, Italy and Greece over the past decade. There are undoubtedly similarities: anger at diminished purchasing power and at the dysfunction of representative democracy; social and political heterogeneity of the protesters, with a significant role played by precarious workers and newcomers to militancy, especially women; occupation of public spaces and utilization of social media; absence of leaders and formal structures, at least in the early phases of these movements. Two factors might nevertheless singularize the French case: the channeling of people's rage against the figure of the President, who has become the symbol of an arrogant and authoritarian neoliberalism, and the country's history of struggles over the social state, which remains part of the collective imaginary.

These hypotheses will need to be confirmed. What can be said with some confidence is that the *gilets jaunes* mobilization constitutes an event in the strong sense of the term—that is, a moment which imposes a temporal rupture in the course of things, with a before and an after. The questioning of social injustice and democratic practices is certainly not new, but it has on this occasion resonated with the population at large, at least in the working class as broadly defined. It has also had interesting effects in the academic world. Rarely have social scientists and social theorists reacted so rapidly to the tumultuous course of events, at the risk of projecting their own desires and expectations, but with the merit of contributing to the collective vibrancy. Two months after the beginning of the movement, three books by multiple authors had already appeared at major publishers.[27] This intellectual effervescence is a signal.

So, too, is the proliferation of debates in all sectors of society. Not unexpectedly, many conservatives are dismissive or suspicious of the *gilets jaunes*, while most progressives are enthralled about their potential to free up a paralyzed social and political system, even if they are aware of the tensions and contradictions within the movement. By claiming that they are the people and by contesting the legitimacy of the elite, the yellow vests are arguably placing themselves in the populist tradition. However, not all populisms are identical. No one knows whether this movement will evolve toward a more recognizable form, but it has at least reminded French politicians of the existence of a category that had disappeared from their vocabulary: *les classes populaires*.

---

[27] Joseph Confavreux, ed., *Le fond de l'air est jaune: Comprendre une révolte inédite*, Paris 2019; Collectif, *'Gilets jaunes': hypothèses sur un mouvement*, Paris 2019; Collectif, *Gilets jaunes: Des clés pour comprendre*, Paris 2018.

new releases from **Haymarket**Books

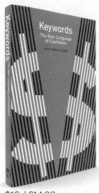

John Patrick Leary
Keywords
The New Language of Capitalism
"If you feel like you're drowning in the endless torrent of capitalist bullshit, turn to this excellent glossary which explains what all those terms really mean. Dip into it, use it as a reference, or read it cover to cover—however you approach it, you'll find it immensely clarifying (and sanity-restoring)."
—Doug Henwood

$16 / £14.99

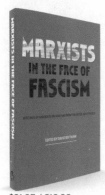

Edited by David Beetham
Marxists in the Face of Fascism
Writings by Marxists on Fascism from the Inter-war Period

An unparalleled documentation of the most important Marxist analyses of fascism and the struggle to resist it.

"Unrivaled and vital . . . allowing us to grasp the major contribution of inter-war Marxism, in its great diversity of theoretical approaches and political orientations "
—Ugo **Palheta**, author *La Possibilité du Fascisme*

$21.95 / £19.99

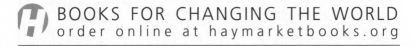

BOOKS FOR CHANGING THE WORLD
order online at haymarketbooks.org

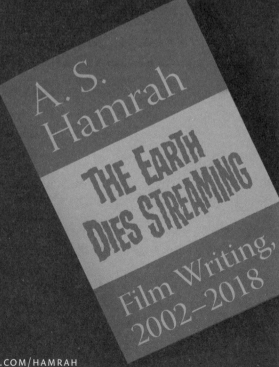

MARK BURTON & PETER SOMERVILLE

DEGROWTH: A DEFENCE

EGROWTH, OR A 'green new deal'? Robert Pollin's contribution to the recent debate on environmental strategy in these pages counterposes the two paths that currently dominate radical discussion of this issue. That they do not exhaust it is clear from the other contributors: Herman Daly, the Grand Old Man of ecological economics, reiterates his call for a 'steady state' economy in his interview with Benjamin Kunkel. Troy Vettese, drawing on the example of the seventeenth century's Little Ice Age, argues for a 'natural geo-engineering project' to lower global temperatures through reforestation, and against mooted artificial geo-engineering solutions, which propose to manipulate the Earth's cloud cover, alter the chemical composition of the oceans or release a 'solar shield' of sunlight-reflecting sulphate particles into the upper atmosphere. At the same time, Mike Davis's discussion of the painstaking archival research by Emmanuel Le Roy Ladurie into the evidence for the Little Ice Age in France illuminates the limits of our knowledge of climate history. What follows will focus on Pollin's trenchant criticisms of degrowth and the version of 'green growth' he offers as an alternative.[1]

Pollin's starting point is the urgent need for emissions reduction to stabilize global temperatures, as set out by the International Panel on Climate Change. Other environmental issues—biodiversity, clean air and water, liveable cities—as well as political questions—social and international equality, for example—are subordinated to the imperative of moderating climate change. 'There are no certainties about what will transpire if we allow the average global temperature to continue rising. But as a basis for action, we only need to understand that there is a non-trivial possibility that the continuation of life on Earth as we know it is at stake.'[2] His programme calls for an extra 1.5–2 per cent of global GDP to be invested annually in a fast-growing programme of clean, non-nuclear, renewable-energy provision, while fossil-fuel industries will be shrunk by 35 per cent over the next twenty years, an annual 2.2 per cent. Taking aim at proponents of degrowth, he argues:

> It is in fact absolutely imperative that some categories of economic activity should now grow massively—those associated with the production and distribution of clean energy. Concurrently, the global fossil-fuel industry needs to contract massively—that is, to 'de-grow' relentlessly over the next forty or fifty years until it has virtually shut down.[3]

This scenario is based on the 'absolute decoupling' of economic growth from fossil-fuel consumption—the former can expand while the latter contracts. Pollin claims this will drive down CO_2 emissions 'by 40 per cent within twenty years, while also supporting rising living standards and expanding job opportunities'. He provides costings for the social support and retraining of fossil-fuel workers: for the US as a whole this amounts to $600 million a year, or 0.2 per cent of the Federal budget. There are no costings for compensating the giant oil, gas and coal corporations; instead, Pollin notes in passing that these behemoths 'will have to be defeated'. Although he concedes the moral case for rich countries to reduce their per capita emissions to the level of poorer ones, he considers it politically unrealistic for the US to do so. Under his programme, US emissions will fall from 16.5 to 5.8 tons per capita after twenty years, but they would still be three times the world average and three times higher than China's per capita emissions, which would fall to 2.3 tons. To compensate, Pollin hopes the US will provide poorer countries with financial help for the transition.

---

[1] Robert Pollin, 'De-growth vs a Green New Deal', NLR 112, July–Aug 2018; Herman Daly and Benjamin Kunkel, 'Ecologies of Scale', NLR 109, Jan–Feb 2018; Troy Vettese, 'To Freeze the Thames', NLR 111, May–June 2018; Mike Davis, 'Taking the Temperature of History', NLR 110, Mar–Apr 2018.
[2] Pollin, 'De-growth vs a Green New Deal', p. 5.
[3] Pollin, 'De-growth vs a Green New Deal', pp. 7–8. The 'degrowth movement' has been organized through the Research & Degrowth network, founded in 2001 by Joan Martinez-Alier (Universitat Autònoma de Barcelona) and Serge Latouche (University of Paris-Sud). Since 2008 it has held biennial international conferences in Paris (2008), Barcelona (2010), Montréal/Venice (2012), Leipzig (2014), Budapest (2016) and Malmö (2018). For an early analysis from this viewpoint, see J. Martinez-Alier, 'Political Ecology, Distributional Conflicts and Economic Incommensurability', NLR I/211, May–June 1995.

Taking issue with Kunkel's opening flourish, that 'fidelity to GDP growth amounts to the religion of the modern world', Pollin counters that, under financialized neoliberalism, the real religion is not growth but maximizing profits 'in order to deliver maximum incomes and wealth for the rich'. While agreeing with the degrowth movement that much global-capitalist production is wasteful and that GDP is a flawed metric, he argues that degrowthers have not produced a viable set of policies to cut greenhouse-gas emissions enough to stabilize global temperatures. Most damningly, it would seem, Pollin charges that degrowth would create soaring levels of poverty and unemployment, while failing to arrest climate change. According to his calculations, a 10 per cent contraction of the global economy, following a degrowth agenda, would create a world-historic slump, with global unemployment rocketing and declining living standards for poor and working-class people, but would still miss IPCC targets.

Limits of decoupling

How well do these claims stand up? Pollin's argument that the drive for profits, not GDP growth, is the real 'religion' of financialized neoliberalism fails to acknowledge that both neoliberalism and financialization are part of capitalism's response to the crisis of profitability that arose following the breakdown of the post-war settlement between capital and labour. The underlying problem is not 'neoliberalism' but the self-expanding system of capitalism, which turns everything into a commodity (real or fictitious), and so threatens the basis for the social and physical reproduction of human society at a variety of levels. Perhaps it is this misidentification of the villain(s)—targeting neoliberalism, not the capitalist mode of production—that helps Pollin to propose what is essentially a social-democratic approach of mitigated capitalism. At the same time, there is no doubt that the imaginary of GDP growth remains a powerful ideological force in its own right, mystifying the real economic processes at stake and instead focusing debate on the idea of expansion as an inherent good. It has a significant influence on decisions regarding production, distribution and consumption, and on the financial system that facilitates each of these elements.

Pollin is partially right to argue that the degrowth movement has not prioritized the formulation of detailed policy proposals on reducing greenhouse-gas emissions; its contributions have generally concentrated on showing how GDP growth makes such reduction harder. However, there are degrowthers who have addressed this question. Kevin Anderson, certainly an ally of degrowth, has proposed a Marshall Plan to decarbonize energy supplies, as well as shifts in 'behaviour and practices' such as frequent flying.[4] Energy and resource caps feature in the work of ecological economist Blake Alcott, for example, and the 'cap and share' variant of this approach has been taken up by Brian Davey and the Irish NGO, FEASTA.[5] Again, Pollin is right to call for a specific sectoral analysis of what needs to happen to make the 'dirty' sectors contract and the clean sectors—the 'replacement economy'—expand. Proponents of degrowth have never argued that *some* sectors should not grow, and shutting down fossil-fuel industries has been a strong strand in their work; it was, for example, the main extra-academic project of the Leipzig degrowth conference in 2014. Crucially, however, this sectoral adjustment needs to take place within an overall envelope that contracts, so that aggregate human activity remains within safe planetary limits and its ecological footprint does not exceed the available biocapacity. This is not just a matter of carbon; it involves water, air, forests, croplands and fishing grounds, as affected by the processes of production, consumption and trade.

Pollin's argument is posited on the 'absolute decoupling' of economic activity from fossil fuels. He rightly emphasizes that the more modest goal of 'relative decoupling'—'through which fossil-fuel consumption and CO2 emissions continue to increase, but at a slower rate than GDP growth'—is not a solution. He goes on to argue that it's fine for economies to continue growing as rapidly as China and India have been doing, so long as the growth process is completely delinked from fossil fuels. However, Pollin doesn't confront the difficulties involved in ensuring that this absolute decoupling will occur. It's implausible that Chinese and Indian growth rates could have been so high *without* soaring fossil-fuel

---

[4] See for example Kevin Anderson, 'Manchester, Paris and 2°C: Laggard or Leader', presentation available on the Greater Manchester Combined Authority website. In the assessment of Anderson and his co-author Alice Bows, 'only the global economic slump has had any significant impact in reversing the trend of rising emissions': 'Beyond "Dangerous" Climate Change: Emission Scenarios for a New World', *Philosophical Transactions of the Royal Society*, vol. 369, no. 1934, 2011.
[5] Blake Alcott, 'Impact Caps: Why Population, Affluence and Technology Strategies Should Be Abandoned', *Journal of Cleaner Production*, vol. 18, no. 6, 2010; Brian Davey, ed., *Sharing for Survival*, Dublin 2012.

consumption—not to mention the carbon emissions caused by changed land-use and the production of concrete and steel. Pollin appeals to a World Resources Institute study which claimed to show that in a number of advanced economies, including the US, Germany and the UK, GDP growth had indeed been decoupled from CO_2 emissions for the period 2000–14.[6] On closer inspection, however, there are serious problems of data quality in the WRI paper, including the use of different reporting protocols by different countries, missing data—emissions from international shipping and aviation are not counted in the national totals, for example—and the 'construct validity' of proxy measures: whether they actually measure what they purport to. The observed effects may reflect one-off or reversible changes—such as the impact of the 2008 economic crisis.[7]

In addition, these supposedly 'decoupling' countries have also been de-industrializing, switching to financialized-capitalist economies with large service sectors, and importing commodities manufactured elsewhere. This creates further problems on both sides of the 'economic growth/carbon emissions' equation. First, through outsourcing production, firms headquartered in the rich countries obtain goods produced at poor-country wage costs, but sold at rich-country consumer-market prices, the sales then figuring in the rich country's GDP.[8] In other words, part of the GDP growth attributed to the supposedly 'decoupling' advanced economies is the result of labour processes in poorer countries. The GDP of rich countries is inflated through this neo-colonial value capture, but the emissions are counted in the emerging economies in which the commodities were produced. This would appear to qualify, if not invalidate, the decoupling claim. The problem is compounded by the fact that the GDP figures enter into both sides of the comparison, since as well as being one of the two variables considered, GDP is used to compute consumption-based emissions which are not directly measured. In any event, the rate of emissions reduction in the apparently decoupling countries would be nowhere near sufficient to avert climate catastrophe.

---

[6] Nate Aden, 'The Roads to Decoupling: 21 Countries Are Reducing Carbon Emissions While Growing GDP', World Resources Institute blog, 5 April 2016.
[7] For a more detailed critique, see Mark Burton, 'New Evidence on Decoupling Carbon Emissions from GDP Growth: What Does It Mean?', Steady State Manchester blog, 15 April 2016.
[8] This is not the only mechanism by which the core countries' income is inflated; transfer pricing by multinationals is another.

As Anderson and Bows have shown, the developed economies—known as 'Annex 1' parties in the Kyoto Accord—need to be cutting emissions at 8 to 10 per cent a year, whereas in the 'decoupling' countries emissions were falling at a mere 2 per cent.[9] Meanwhile, global emissions for the period 2000–14 actually increased by 45 per cent, with the world economy as a whole showing no signs of decoupling. Pollin therefore risks underestimating the rate of emissions reduction required to avoid catastrophic climate change.

Moreover, when the full picture of material flows through national economies is considered—the 'physical throughput' emphasized by Herman Daly—it turns out that there is no decoupling at all between resource use and GDP growth.[10] While Pollin is right to emphasize carbon emissions, it's also clear that present levels of production-consumption (let alone their growth) require materials which are, to varying extents, becoming scarcer.[11] The cost of obtaining them has risen, putting a growing strain on the global economy—the dynamic that underpinned the *Limits to Growth* business-as-usual scenario, with its system crash in the mid twenty-first century. Their extraction entails the destruction of livelihoods and ecosystems across the world, and particularly in the global South. All this would seem to put degrowth firmly back on the agenda, since to achieve a radical reduction in emissions we need a global economy that is considerably smaller in material terms.[12]

The scale of the world economy exceeds the Earth's biological and physical capacity to absorb the impacts and restore the resources used. The Global Footprint Network currently estimates humankind's collective material footprint at 1.7 times the available biocapacity. Daly is correct to argue that population size is an important part of environmental

[9] Anderson and Bows, 'Beyond "Dangerous" Climate Change'.

[10] Thomas Wiedmann, Heinz Schandl et al., 'The Material Footprint of Nations', *Proceedings of the National Academy of Sciences*, vol. 112, no. 20, May 2015. See Daly and Kunkel, 'Ecologies of Scale', p. 89.

[11] Carlos de Castro, Margarita Mediavilla et al., 'Global Wind Power Potential: Physical and Technological Limits', *Energy Policy*, vol. 39, no. 10, October 2011; 'Global Solar Electric Potential: A Review of Their Technical and Sustainable Limits', *Renewable and Sustainable Energy Reviews*, vol. 28, December 2013.

[12] Post-extractivism—the movement against extractivism in the global South—has been closely allied with degrowth. See Alberto Acosta, 'Post-Growth and Post-Extractivism: Two Sides of the Same Cultural Transformation', *Alternautas*, March 2016; Alberto Acosta and Ulrich Brand, *Salidas del laberinto capitalista: Decrecimiento y postextractivismo*, Barcelona 2017.

impact.[13] However, while global emissions are still rising, the rate of population growth has slowed significantly—increasing from 4 billion to 7 billion between 1975 and 2010, but only projected to reach 8 billion by the mid-2020s and around 9 billion by 2050.[14] The main driver of the slow-down is the declining rate of fertility, already below replacement level in Europe, though higher in India and sub-Saharan Africa. Historically, rising living standards, urbanization and education, particularly for women, have been associated with falling fertility, while poorer and more unequal countries tend to have higher rates. If these conditions were tackled, and primary health care as well as modern contraception made freely available, the global population could stabilize and even begin to decline before 2050.

Green expansion?

What of Pollin's proposal to stabilize the climate by investing an annual 2 per cent of global GDP in clean energy? His argument is that this switch to renewables can cut global emissions by 40 per cent within twenty years 'while also supporting rising living standards and expanding job opportunities'. So far, however, the expansion of renewables has come as an addition to fossil-fuel supplies, rather than as a replacement for them (see Table 1, overleaf). The countries that are most advanced in developing renewable energy, such as Denmark and Germany, have also expanded their consumption of fossil fuels, particularly coal; the same applies to the US, China, India, Canada and Australia. To replace oil, coal and gas with other sources of energy would take something like an 18-fold increase in renewables deployment, at current levels of energy consumption. If worldwide energy usage were to increase, as Pollin indicates, then the challenge would be even greater.

The contradiction of the 'green new deal' is that GDP growth makes reducing emissions far harder. Expanding the economy inevitably

---

[13] 'Environmental impact is the product of the number of people times per capita resource use': 'Ecologies of Scale', p. 93.

[14] Projections beyond 2050 involve a high degree of uncertainty. In a 2014 paper Patrick Gerland and his colleagues estimate a global population between 9.6 and 12.3 billion in 2100. See Gerland et al., 'World Population Stabilization Unlikely this Century', *Science*, vol. 346, no. 6206, 10 October 2014; see also K. C. Samir and Wolfgang Lutz, 'The Human Core of the Shared Socioeconomic Pathways: Population Scenarios by Age, Sex and Level of Education for All Countries to 2100', *Global Environmental Change*, vol. 42, January 2017, pp. 181–92.

TABLE I: *Primary Energy Consumption by Fuel, Million Tonne Equivalents*

	1970	1980	1990	2000	2010	2020
Oil	2,253	2,986	3,153	3,580	4,021	4,564
Gas	890	1,291	1,767	2,182	2,874	3,534
Coal	1,483	1,813	2,246	2,385	3,636	3,697
Nuclear	18	161	453	584	626	674
Hydro	266	385	487	601	779	1,015
Renewables	2	7	35	59	234	794
Total	4,912	6,642	8,142	9,390	12,170	14,278

Source: BP Energy Outlook, 2018.

means more extraction, production, distribution and consumption, and each of these processes produces emissions. If Pollin's renewable-energy investment plan also succeeded in generating tens of millions of new jobs and raising living standards worldwide, as he hopes, that would mean a further increase in the consumption of carbon-intensive services and products—unless the relevant industries were thoroughly decarbonized, probably in conjunction with caps on energy use, extraction and land-use conversion.

In theory, contracting the world economy need not hurt the relatively poor, since high emissions are strongly correlated with concentrations of wealth and income: globally, the top 10 per cent of emitters contribute approximately 45 per cent of greenhouse-gas emissions, while the bottom 50 per cent contribute only 13 per cent.[15] Deep economic retrenchment can be managed equitably, as was demonstrated during the hardship of the Special Period in Cuba in the early 90s, when punitive US sanctions exacerbated the impact of the collapse of the Soviet Union. The possibility that contraction might take place in a properly democratic fashion was explored by André Gorz—acclaimed as a forerunner by the degrowth movement—who called for forms of workers' self-management as a

[15] Lucas Chancel and Thomas Piketty, 'Carbon and Inequality from Kyoto to Paris: Trends in the Global Inequality of Carbon Emissions (1998–2013) and Prospects for an Equitable Adaptation Fund', Paris School of Economics, November 2015, p. 50.

means to 'restore the correlation between less work and less consumption, on one hand, and more autonomy and more existential security on the other'.[16] Pollin's proposals for a 'just transition' to renewable energy that would also contribute to greater global equity are welcome; but so far work in this area, including Pollin's, has tended to concentrate on the fossil-fuel industry.[17]

Finally, Pollin argues that a degrowth agenda to shrink global GDP by 10 per cent over the next twenty years would entail a slump four times deeper than the 2008 recession, with world unemployment soaring amid steep spending cuts, yet the net effect would be to push CO_2 emissions down by a mere 10 per cent—from 32 to 29 billion tons—nowhere near the necessary fall to 20 billion tons by 2040. This is correct. On its own, managed economic contraction—which isn't the same as degrowth, but is a component of it—will not bring about the kind of emissions cuts we need. But as we have seen, maintaining aggregate expansion of the economy, tracked by GDP growth, will add to the hill that has to be climbed. Besides, even the elimination of fossil fuels may not be enough to ensure the future of life on Earth, given the increasing pressures on ecosystems and scarce resources. Capitalism's relentless quest for new forms of profit-making, and for natural resources to exploit and extract, is not limited to oil, coal and gas.

Even if this is not on the cards in the immediate future, an ecologically sustainable world economy would have to be delinked from the drive for profits, and ordered instead around the principle of deploying human capabilities to meet human needs, within the limits of Earth's biocapacity. In other words, it would be a socialist mode of production of some sort. This would need to involve the equitable control and reduction of the material scale of the global economy, together with targeted curtailment of emissions.[18] That means drastic action to cut industrial production (of goods that are not needed, that involve high energy consumption, that

---

[16] André Gorz, 'Political Ecology: Expertocracy versus Self-Limitation', NLR I/202, Nov–Dec 1993; see also *Ecology as Politics*, London 1987.

[17] See the examples of local outcomes for energy workers in Europe, China, Australia, Argentina and the US cited in Anabella Rosenberg, 'Strengthening Just Transition Policies in International Climate Governance', Stanley Foundation, Muscatine, IA 2017.

[18] Decreasing the scale of the global material economy is proposed here as a means to an end, emissions reduction—a necessary condition for strong sustainability. Arguably, this voluntary downscaling, one dimension of degrowth, may be a desirable end in itself.

do not last) as well as industrial construction (roads, airports, speculative skyscrapers and shopping malls), industrial agriculture (fossil-fuel dependent monocultures that destroy soils and water supplies, and require huge energy inputs to bring food to the table) and industrial distribution (sea, air and road transportation systems, all highly dependent on fossil-fuel combustion). The working week would be much shorter, and consumption in the developed world, and by elites in the developing world, severely circumscribed. Heating would be provided entirely by electricity generated from renewable sources. Transport would largely be public, powered by electricity or hydrogen fuel cells. Construction would no longer involve the use of cement or steel. Agriculture would be guided by the principles of agroecology: biodiversity and complexity as the foundation for soil quality, plant health and crop productivity; diversified farming practices, including crop rotation, polycultures, agroforestry, green manures, crop-livestock mixtures, cover crops and mulching.[19]

None of this suggests that it would be easy to steer the world economy towards its ecologically consistent size. Indeed, it perhaps hardly seems likely that this will happen. Yet that does not mean there is any escape from the fundamental problem that the global economy now far exceeds the capacity of Earth's systems to sustain its demands; expanding it further can only make matters worse. The mitigated capitalism of a 'green new deal' will be little help, because it leaves the overall system of commodification, and the motors of expansion, firmly in place. How degrowth might happen we don't know. A fortuitous combination of popular struggle and collapse of the capitalist system is perhaps the only route. That isn't to say that good governmental action, including investment in clean energy and demand-reduction measures, can't help. But for it to work, government policy would have to break from its normal mode of handmaiden to global capital. Unrealistic? Implausible? Probably, but no more than Pollin's imaginary of green accumulation to the rescue.

---

[19] Third World Network, *Agroecology: Key Concepts, Principles and Practices*, Penang and Berkeley 2015.

LOLA SEATON

GREEN QUESTIONS

A S TIME ROLLS on and the IPCC's deadlines for reducing the rise in global temperatures get closer, the prospect of climate catastrophe looms larger, and the problem of how to avert it becomes ever more pressing. This is the question that has been under discussion in recent numbers of NLR. The debate has featured interventions from a number of distinct positions, on both sides of the Atlantic and across different political generations. Herman Daly, a pioneer in the field of ecological economics, was quizzed on his programme for a steady-state system by Benjamin Kunkel, *n+1* founding editor and author of *Buzz*. Canadian environmental historian Troy Vettese argued for a pollution-shrinking 'half-earth' project of natural geo-engineering and eco-austerity. Taking the opposite tack, the radical economist Robert Pollin called for massive global investment in renewable energy. In the current number, UK-based scholar-activists Mark Burton and Peter Somerville reply with a defence of 'degrowth'. Still to come are contributions from an eco-feminist perspective and from the global South.[1]

At this mid-point in the debate, it may be helpful to pause and take stock. As well as putting forward their own solutions, the contributors have responded—sometimes with assent, but often in the form of rebuttals or correctives—to each other's. The result of this direct engagement is that, reading the texts in sequence, one feels one has witnessed a conversation. Yet, in a conversation stretched across twelve months and congealed in text, the latest voices can become the loudest—having both the opportunity to respond to everything that has come before, and the privilege of going temporarily unanswered. So, in order to collect one's thoughts on the debate so far—to reflect on the progress made, the problems thrown up, the questions still untabled—it may be worth, as it were, putting the thinkers in a room together, to help the existing strands of dialogue become more audible.

Sacrifice?

One way of comparing the contributions is to regard them as providing different answers to the question: what does the world need to cut in order to avoid global disaster? Herman Daly defines 'environmental impact' as 'the product of the number of people times per capita resource use'. Following the logic of this equation, Daly thinks we need to reduce our use of resources, including, but not limited to, fossil fuels, and to limit population growth. To implement these reductions, he envisions some kind of cap-and-trade system. In the case of resources, there would be a 'limit on the right to deplete what you own', and that right would be purchasable 'by auction from the government'. In the case of population, everyone would be given the right to reproduce once, but since not everyone can, or wants to have children, those rights could be reallocated 'by sale or by gift'. Daly also advocates a minimum and maximum income. These redistributive policies are critical accompaniments to his caps on resource use and population growth since without setting a limit on inequality too, the distribution of the rights to consume and to have children could be drastically uneven and unfair (the mega-rich could, for example, monopolize reproduction).

Taking land scarcity as the 'fundamental metric' for his 'alternative green political economy', Troy Vettese's 'eco-austere' answer is that we must reduce our energy consumption and cut out meat and dairy. Mandatory veganism would free up farmland for 'land-hungry' clean-energy infrastructure like wind turbines and solar panels, which could then become the world's primary way of meeting its energy needs. The extra land could also be used for natural geo-engineering projects like large-scale rewilding ('half-earthing') to create ecosystems that would act as carbon sinks.

---

[1] Herman Daly, 'Ecologies of Scale: Interview by Benjamin Kunkel', NLR 109, Jan–Feb 2018; Troy Vettese, 'To Freeze the Thames: Natural Geo-Engineering and Biodiversity', NLR 111, May–June 2018; Robert Pollin, 'De-Growth vs a Green New Deal', NLR 112, July–August 2018; Mark Burton and Peter Somerville, 'Degrowth: A Defence', NLR 115, Jan–Feb 2019.

Robert Pollin takes issue with Vettese's 'fundamental metric': he thinks Vettese's estimates about how much land renewable-energy systems would require are inflated. With land scarcity not a limiting factor in Pollin's account, cutting our energy consumption—beyond reducing energy wastage—becomes unnecessary. So, unlike Daly and Vettese, Pollin is almost exclusively concerned with reducing not energy use but fossil-fuel use: 'To make real progress on climate stabilization, the single most critical project is to cut the consumption of oil, coal and natural gas dramatically and without delay.' Through concerted global investment in both clean-energy infrastructure and more energy-efficient 'technologies and practices', we can cut out fossil fuels while continuing to 'achieve the same, or higher, levels of energy service'.

In the latest contribution to the debate, published in this issue, Mark Burton and Peter Somerville agree with Pollin about the necessity for 'targeted curtailment of [carbon] emissions' through a transition to clean energy. But, whereas Pollin is wary about the political and economic viability of massively shrinking the economy—which he fears could result in 'a green great depression', featuring impossibly high unemployment and unacceptable drops in living standards—Burton and Somerville argue that a drastic contraction of the material size of the economy through cutting industrial production, construction, agriculture and distribution is the essential complement to a switch to renewables. They calculate that to generate enough energy at current usage levels without recourse to oil, coal or natural gas would require 'an 18-fold increase in renewables deployment', and so argue that if energy consumption were to increase further—as it would if economic activity continues to expand—weaning ourselves off fossil fuels would only be more difficult.

Pollin's answer stands out from the rest because his version of the transition to clean energy would mostly not be felt by individual consumers, whose energy use, unaffected by the change of provenance in quantitative terms, could continue as normal. This prompts a second question that may throw the specificity of Pollin's contribution into relief: how much sacrifice do the different proposed cuts require? However costly Pollin's proposals—he estimates they would suck up 'between 1.5 and 2 per cent of global GDP every year', which amounts to roughly $1 trillion—and however temporarily painful the transition (necessary job losses in fossil-fuel industries, which would need to be cushioned by adequate social provision including retraining and relocating workers), the question of sacrifice in Pollin's text is largely out of frame.[2] By using different energy resources, and using them better, we don't have to use less energy; we can even use more. Far from climate change 'changing everything',[3] as long as 'energy consumption, and economic activity more generally' are '*absolutely decoupled* from the consumption of fossil fuels', both can go on as before. The key, repeated figure in Pollin's proposal sounds small—a mere 1.5 per cent—whilst the scale of the projected changes is huge—global and industrial, even supra-industrial. This combination makes their human cost seem at once negligible and abstract. Predominantly affecting large-scale industries and to be handled by remote global bureaucracies, Pollin's solutions release us from significantly altering our lifestyles and call for little cur-tailment of individual freedom.

Vettese's solutions, by contrast, deprive everyone of meat and require many people in the world to use *a lot* less energy, especially Americans, who would have to reduce their energy consumption by more than 80 per cent: currently the average US citizen uses about 12,000 watts per day, whereas in Vettese's eco-austere society each person would use no more than 2,000. Though neither local nor small in scale ('half-earthing'), Vettese's proposals feature behavioural changes at the level of the individual, and he makes no secret of the relative hardship these changes might entail ('eco-austerity'). Though Pollin mentions job losses and a 'just transition', his emphasis is on net job creation, and our imaginations are not seriously engaged in thinking through the personal loss and upheaval that would surely accompany the elimina-tion of whole industries.

Daly's proposals provide something of a bridge between Pollin's technology-enabled unlimited consumption and Vettese's non-optional austerity. In Daly's steady state, the rights to deplete resources and to

---

[2] The latest issue of *n+1* expresses approval for Pollin's approach precisely by suggesting that the question of sacrifice in green debates is misplaced: 'The most radical and hopeful response to climate change shouldn't be, What do we give up?', but 'How do we collectively improve our overall quality of life? It is a wel-fare question, one that has less to do with consumer choices—like changing light bulbs—than with the spending of trillions and trillions of still-available dollars on decoupling economic growth and wealth from carbon-based fuels and carbon-intensive products, including plastics': 'The Intellectual Situation: The Best of a Bad Situation', *n+1*, no. 33, Winter 2019, p. 8.
[3] Naomi Klein, *This Changes Everything*, Harmondsworth 2014, p. 4.

populate the world are both exchangeable. This means that the inverse deprivations can be traded too: the seller of a right is buying an obligation to make a sacrifice—though, crucially, this may not feel like a sacrifice (the seller of their right to reproduce may not want children). Cushioning the iron fist of state-mandated sacrifice is thus the glove of flexibility in terms of how that sacrifice is distributed: using the organizational genius of the market, privileges and privations would be allocated according to individual need and personal choice. This is why Daly is fond of cap-and-trade systems: they combine aggregate control—over the total amount of carbon we collectively emit or the total number of children born—with as much personal autonomy as is compatible with such macro-restrictions.[4]

Pollin's appeal

Pollin's proposal stands apart in a more general way because it has a kind of *prima facie* plausibility that the others lack. Its exclusion of the necessity of permanent personal sacrifice no doubt accounts for much of this impression. Particularly in the US—with its almost fanatical enshrinement of freedom, particularly the freedom to consume and to acquire property—it is hard to imagine either Daly or Vettese's policies, let alone those of Burton and Somerville, gaining much traction. Intuitively one suspects that the consumption habits of American citizens—whether meat-eating or car-driving—would be tough to crack.[5] Daly's wealth restrictions seem perhaps more quixotic than his ecological ones. During the interview, Kunkel reports that, anecdotally, Daly's population proposal is the one that people tend to 'find most difficult to contemplate', but the prospect of America's oligarchic governing

---

[4] Vettese, on the other hand, is sceptical about the efficacy of cap-and-trade systems. 'The world's biggest cap-and-trade programme for CO2 emissions, the European Emissions Trading System (ETS), has largely functioned to forestall meaningful action', he argues, since prices are kept deliberately low to placate industry by ensuring the impact is trivial. To be effective, Daly's cap-and-trade systems would need to 'address the problem of the class capture of markets'.

[5] J. R. McNeill suggests obduracy—led by the US— was very much the tone at the UN environmental conference held in Rio de Janeiro in 1992: 'The Americans made it clear that US "lifestyles" were not up for negotiation. Other countries matched this stance.' See his *Something New Under the Sun: An Environmental History of the Twentieth-Century World*, Harmondsworth 2000, p. 355. But the intransigence of UN delegates is not just about protecting consumerist 'lifestyles', but livelihoods, and reflects the fragile situation of ordinary people, who often can't afford to compromise as they struggle to sustain themselves in conditions of rising inequality.

class overseeing the implementation of Daly's maximum income seems almost more unthinkable.

Pollin's exclusion of sacrifice also appeals because it speaks to the scepticism some feel about the efficacy of small-scale, individual efforts to reduce humankind's ecological footprint. Unlike households switching to greener light bulbs or avoiding plastic-wrapped goods, the global scale of Pollin's suggestions seems adequate to the size of the problem.[6] His programme is attractive from certain angles on account of its narrow focus, too. Daly and Vettese's contributions include multiple policies—depletion quotas *and* population caps, or veganism *and* reduced consumption—and their concerns are several and broader. Pollin's exclusive concern is fossil fuels. His logic is streamlined: burning fossil fuels 'is responsible for generating about 74 per cent of overall global greenhouse gas emissions';[7] greenhouse gases warm the planet; therefore the most direct and immediate way to stabilize global temperatures is to stop burning fossil fuels. Past effective environmental action—against ozone-destroying CFCs for example—suggests that single-issue, or single-substance initiatives, which attract public support more easily and are more conducive to targeted legislation, have a greater chance of success.

All the other contributors express concerns that go beyond fossil fuels, including ecological ones: both Daly and Burton and Somerville are interested in depletable natural resources other than those carbon-based ones we can turn into energy, whilst Vettese is concerned for biodiversity, which, he argues, 'needs to be upheld' not just because it increases carbon retention, but 'in its own right'. In Pollin's more anthropocentric contribution, by contrast, in which global warming is the sole focus, nature features only as an economic category, a potential energy resource; its existence is scarcely imagined outside of its human use.

The other contributions contain extra-ecological reflections, too, or carry extra-ecological implications—social, economic and political ones about

---

[6] George Monbiot has argued that even well-intentioned citizens need governments to regulate their ecological behaviour for them because 'self-enforced abstinence is both ineffective' and 'unattractive': 'Environmental Feedback: A Reply to Clive Hamilton', NLR 45, May–June 2007, p. 113.

[7] Robert Pollin, 'Global Green Growth for Human Development', UNDP Human Development Report, 2016, p. 3.

how we could organize ourselves better and more fairly, and particularly about whether continuing to produce and circulate increasing quantities of commodities constitutes a social good. Though prompted by the climate crisis, these questions about value and fairness nevertheless exceed it. Other than Pollin—who admits current consumption can be 'wasteful', but doesn't advocate setting limits on it—all the contributors are critical of the amount we consume. But these criticisms frequently stem from concerns that go beyond sustainability. Vettese, for example, approvingly quotes Alyssa Battistoni's reflections on how converting to a 'climate-stable future' might be an opportunity to re-think which kinds of work are truly socially useful and improve people's lives 'without consuming vast amounts of resources'. Likewise, Burton and Somerville at one point suggest 'voluntary downscaling' of the material economy might be 'a desirable end in itself'.

This extra-ecological critique of the untrammelled consumption on which economic expansion depends is most pronounced in the interview with Daly, who, in Kunkel's words, believes 'that life, or a society, ought to have some purpose beyond economic growth'. Kunkel suggests that some of Daly's readers—though not Kunkel himself—'detect a certain religious orientation' in this notion that societies ought to be guided by more enlightened values than mere enthusiasm for material increase. Whether or not we agree in calling this conviction 'religious'—perhaps it is to the extent that it replaces the 'fidelity to GDP' which Kunkel dubs the modern world's religion (about which more below)—it is not an *economic* rationale for degrowth, nor, significantly, an exclusively ecological one. Endless expansion may well not be ecologically sustainable, but the suggestion here is that even if it were, it would still not be desirable—on other, extra-ecological grounds. This is not an objection to the environmental havoc unlimited growth wreaks, but to its meaninglessness, and a call to stop being carried away by its autotelic pretensions.

Pollin's text is distinctive for its relative silence on these matters. Giving his single-minded attention to how we generate energy and how well, rather than how much, we use it, he does not articulate a broader socioeconomic vision within which his global clean-energy programme might fit. Daly's existential meditations on human purpose and his concerns about wealth distribution barely enter Pollin's text, such is its tactical, dedicated focus on renewables. In the short passage where Pollin does discuss the possibility of introducing measures that would equalize emissions between rich, high-emitting countries and their poorer, low-emitting counterparts, he is categorical: yes, Americans emit far more carbon per capita than anyone else, and yes, they have been doing so for the past century, but—as for measures preventing US citizens from emitting more than the rest of the world, measures for which Pollin acknowledges there is 'a solid ethical case'—'there is absolutely no chance that they will be implemented', and 'we do not have the luxury to waste time on huge global efforts fighting for unattainable goals'.

Strategy in the second sense

Pollin dismisses these social and ethical questions on the grounds of political realism, abetted by a sense of urgency. He thinks it is 'more constructive' to concentrate on specific, concrete goals, than to 'present broad generalities about the nature of economic growth, positive or negative'. Pollin's strategic reticence about problems of value and fairness, coupled with his insistent single-mindedness, is part of what makes his text persuasive at one level—and distinctive, since Pollin's pragmatism, and his seeming certainty about the limits of the politically possible ('absolutely no chance'), is largely missing from the other contributions. This series, as its title suggests, is about strategy; its emphasis, as Pollin points out, is on 'what is to be done'. But the question of how to avert planetary disaster is not just a question calling for prescriptive technical strategies that examine the efficacy and priority of green technologies and behaviours, and imagine future, greener scenarios. It is also a question about *political* strategy, which calls for descriptive analysis of the present moment, and for attempts to identify what kind of political obstacles sit in the way of implementing those technical solutions at the required speed and with the necessary thoroughness, with a view to asking how those obstacles might be overcome.

We have little trouble envisaging greener futures—wind turbines, solar panels, afforestation and so on—but what we mostly don't seem to know is the answer to this second question about how to get from here to there, or, in Daly's words, to map the route between 'how things are' and 'how things ought to be'. This question is hugely complicated, and is left to different degrees unanswered in all the contributions—including Pollin's, despite his ostensible shrewdness. The absence is most conspicuous in the interview with Daly, where Kunkel gently presses him on it. Distrustful of historical materialism, Daly fails to provide any alternative theory of what motors historical change, and of who or what would secure the uptake of his policies, except through 'an appeal to morality, whether that's sufficient or not'. Discussing the political unfeasibility of his population policy, he says his instinct is to 'back off the idea', 'because people just don't want it. I'm not a dictator. I just present this as an idea. If one day people come to the realization that it's necessary to limit total population', then, he challenges, 'show me a better way'. Daly rejects the philosopher-king role: his conception of his intellectual task is to think up methods for achieving goals, but the problem of winning public support for them is left to others. He is an economist, not a political scientist, and not an activist, and certainly 'not a dictator'; politics will catch up with him—or it won't ('sufficient or not'). In the absence of more robust theorizing about how this hypothetical change would come about—except through mass epiphanic conversion—Daly's policies risk political irrelevance, since we are left without any meaningful sense of how they would come to seem necessary to the people in a position to implement them. The same could apply to Vettese; Burton and Somerville, too.

Impersonating 'a sort of doctrinaire Marxist for a moment', Kunkel explores this limit of Daly's thinking: 'Engels might say that your steady-state economy is too utopian' since 'you don't specify a material or "scientific" historical process that would effect the change.' Daly says he doesn't 'believe the story of determinism'. This prompts Kunkel to ask: 'You don't believe it because you think ethical, moral, religious conversions do have a material effect on how things happen?' 'Yes', Daly replies. 'Purpose is causative in the world. If it is not, then we should all go back to sleep.'

What exactly is 'purpose', for Daly? People have all kinds of purposes, and they need not be ethical (and ethical purposes may not win out). The desire to make a profit could be construed as a kind of purpose; it is certainly causative.[8] Daly seems to exclude these callous kinds of motivation, since he has in mind purposes 'beyond economic growth'. Nonetheless, his striking statement—'Purpose is causative'—in a sense crystallizes this failure—not Daly's alone—to address the question of

---

[8] Although perhaps profit-making, however consciously willed, is not best described as a 'purpose' since it is not so much a subjective desire as an objective requirement of the capitalist system—the way aiming to win a race is not really a personal motivation, but more like a premise of participating.

political strategy. 'Purpose' is an abstraction, floating free of any specific historical actors, and one senses that its predicate, 'causative'—an unusual adjectival rendering of the more familiar noun or verb from which it is derived—is a slight grammatical evasion, which allows Daly to avoid saying 'purpose causes'—a claim that sounds more conspicuously metaphysical and unsubstantiated. Which purposes, and whose, prove causative, Daly doesn't specify. This is a species of idealism, semi-concealed by grammar, and it induces scepticism even as it elicits sympathy: moral awakenings may have material consequences, but they do not necessarily outweigh the causativeness of the purposes of, for example, the coal lobby.

But Pollin, too, despite being less starry-eyed about the power of do-gooders, and generally more politically worldly (his jargonistic phrase 'climate-stabilization imperative' is characteristic in this respect), fails to specify how the intergovernmental global bureaucracy his investment plan presumably requires would obtain enough political clout to override the interests of the fossil-fuel industries. Pollin raises this issue only to swiftly drop it:

> Of course, both privately owned fossil-fuel companies, such as Exxon-Mobil and Chevron, and publicly owned companies like Saudi Aramco and Gazprom have massive interests at stake in preventing reductions in fossil-fuel consumption; they also wield enormous political power. These powerful vested interests will have to be defeated.

Pollin straight away moves on, passing over the question of precisely how the interests of these powerful, extremely wealthy industries are to be overcome. Pollin's passive construction—'to be defeated'—is symptomatic of his leaving this question unanswered.

Growth as such

In his introduction to the interview with Daly, Kunkel wrote, as we saw, that 'fidelity to GDP amounts to the religion of the modern world'. These innocent words caused a small storm. Everyone weighed in with their thoughts on whether increasing GDP is in fact essential to contemporary capitalist societies (which became a *de facto* synonym for 'the modern world'), and, if so, whether this is a result, as Kunkel's claim implies, of the 'ideological' sway it holds (as a 'religion'), or whether growth is an internal economic necessity reducible to the logic of capital.

Vettese takes issue with both parts of Kunkel's remark, reminding us, firstly, that GDP is just an 'abstract measurement', and as such 'mere foam' to 'what goes on in the [economy's] churning depths', and secondly, that growth is not a 'religion' insofar as it is not, primarily, occasioned by an ideological devotion to what measures it. What drives capitalist economies and motors their perpetual expansions is not a collective theoretical commitment to increasing their size, but individual producers' unrelenting compulsion to make ever-increasing profits. This is not an optional matter, and it is in some significant sense not a subjective one, but a 'structural imperative'. Vettese implies it is Kunkel's mistake to suggest that GDP also motivates the expansion it quantifies.

Though sticking with Kunkel's word 'religion' rather than Vettese's de-ideologized and depersonalized 'structural imperative', Pollin agrees with Vettese that 'the real religion' of the modern world—at least of the world since 'neoliberalism became the predominant economic-policy model' in the mid 70s—is not growth, but 'maximizing profits for business in order to deliver maximum incomes and wealth for the rich'. And devotees of these gods of profit-making, Pollin tells us, mostly pay little heed to growth. The massive concentration of wealth effected by neoliberal policies has in fact come at the expense of growth in the advanced economies, the average rate of which has fallen to less than half that sustained during the *trente glorieuses*.

Burton and Somerville are in agreement with Vettese's initial correction that GDP is the 'foam' to the churning 'depths' of profit-making, and—echoing Vettese's spatial metaphor—argue that growth is driven by the accumulation of capital in private hands, and so fixating on GDP risks missing this underlying reality. Yet, shifting their weight slightly to take Kunkel's part, Burton and Somerville also emphasize GDP's importance on the ideological plane, and insist, against Vettese, that it is an influential 'cultural notion', which has a determining effect on economic behaviour: 'growth remains a powerful ideological force in its own right', which focuses 'debate on the idea of expansion as an inherent good'.

Burton and Somerville stress the material economic effects of this GDP 'imaginary': it 'has a significant influence on decisions regarding production, distribution and consumption'. But growth fetishism does not only affect the running of the economy; it also influences electoral politics. The stamp of economic ascendancy, a steadily increasing GDP is also a prerequisite for electoral success, and failure to achieve it is punished at the polls. An expanding economy and rising living standards are what consuming citizens in advanced economies expect, and it is what politicians in capitalist liberal democracies must promise to secure majorities. The *sine qua non* of electoral viability, growth is thus not just a self-activating outcome of capitalism's drive for profit, but the ideological cornerstone of its social legitimacy. Or, to borrow two of Michael Mann's pithy formulations: 'GDP growth is why capitalism is seen as a great success story', whilst 'political success is actually measured by economic growth'.[9]

Yet growth is not just a fetish of politicians; that fetish reflects the perceived desires of the consumers who vote for them. Mann reminds us of this dynamic when he writes that 'the political treadmill is not imposed by states on unwilling subjects, for these measure their own success by material consumption, and they will support politicians who they think will deliver this.'[10] This would suggest that if giving up growth is to become electorally viable, the electorate needs to enable politicians to give up their promise to deliver it, which means consumer-voters giving up their expectations of increasing affluence, or finding other ways to 'measure their own success'.

But if GDP is the electorate's 'religion', it is also, as Vettese says, just an 'abstract measurement', so when people believe in GDP, what is it, specifically, that they are believing in? That is, when people demand growth, what is the content of their demand? Perhaps 'material consumption', as Mann suggests, but only if by this he is not simply talking about the latest Apple gadgets but those consumer goods—like food and shelter and central heating—essential to a decent quality of life. In that case, to believe in growth is to subscribe to the notion—capitalism's historic self-justification, famously captured in the slogan 'what's good for General Motors is good for America'—that sustaining profitability for private companies is ultimately a public good because it leads to higher living standards. Then one could see GDP as something like the symbolic marker of capitalism's putative conversion of 'private vices' into 'public benefits'.[11] This is where Daly's critique of GDP as

---

[9] Michael Mann, *The Sources of Social Power: Globalizations, 1954–2011*, vol. 4, New York 2013, pp. 325, 365.
[10] Mann, *The Sources of Social Power*, p. 364.

an empirical measure becomes relevant. He argues that this connection between profit and welfare—a connection institutionalized by GDP—hardly holds: 'the coupling of GDP and welfare is loose, or even non-existent beyond some sufficiency threshold.' A figure that records how much we collectively produce and consume does not tell us much about our quality of life.

As Pollin points out, self-sustaining growth is no longer a reality in capitalist economies in the West. This is the fact with which Robert Brenner begins his introduction to the inaugural issue of *Catalyst*: 'The capitalist system long ago lost the capacity to realize its ostensible historic comparative advantage and justification—to drive unceasing capital accumulation, which makes for self-sustaining economic growth and creates the potential for rising living standards.' But Brenner goes further than Pollin, and suggests that as growth has slowed, so has people's belief in it. 'In the last thirty years or so', as 'upward redistribution' of wealth has increasingly replaced its production, even the notion that higher private profits lead to higher living standards has lost its purchase on the public imaginary: the 'cliché has ceased to hold—and the world's capitalist classes no longer really proclaim it'.[12] Brenner suggests that people no longer take seriously the idea that there is a necessary connection between increased company profits and enhanced social well-being. According to Brenner's account, it is not just the rate of growth that is in decline, but the ideological aura surrounding it.

Degrees of capitalism

Pollin seems to partly subscribe to this view insofar as he takes the former to be a kind of proof of the latter: growth has stagnated since the onset of neoliberalism; this indicates that the capitalist classes have other priorities (profits). But Burton and Somerville offer an alternative understanding of financialized neoliberalism, which, they suggest, was 'capitalism's response to the crisis of profitability' that ensued after the postwar boom. In other words, neoliberal policies—including massive deregulation of a surging financial sector—were not expressions of some GDP-spurning mutation of the capitalist system whereby the desire

---

[11] These phrases are Wolfgang Streeck's. See his 'How Will Capitalism End?', NLR 87, May–June 2014.
[12] The Editors, 'Introducing Catalyst', *Catalyst*, vol. 1, no. 1, Spring 2017.

to amass extreme private wealth suddenly overshadowed the growth imperative, but were rather symptoms of an ongoing commitment to that imperative insofar as they represent capitalism's improvised reaction to the falling rate of return on productive investment.

Burton and Somerville complete their criticism by wondering whether Pollin's 'misidentification of the villain(s)'—his blaming financialized neoliberalism and thus the stagnation of growth, rather than growth itself—is what allows him to make ecological proposals that operate essentially within 'mitigated capitalism'. They suggest that by implying a distinction between forms of capitalism—a mid-twentieth-century, less maleficent variety, and the contemporary, 'unleashed', neoliberal kind—Pollin can associate a welfare-enhancing and ecologically sensible version of growth with the former, and the bastardization of these values with the comparatively anaemic growth rates of only the most recent iterations of capitalism.

It is perhaps no coincidence that Daly, the other contributor whose proposals ostensibly operate within the prevailing mode of production, also wants to insist on the idea of degrees of capitalism: 'Capitalism in the sense of financialized monopoly capitalism, geared towards continuous growth and concentration of incomes, is really bad', but it also has less terrible incarnations: a 'small-scale capitalism, operating within scale and distributive limits'. By making such evaluative distinctions, Daly can adumbrate a better angel of capitalism—associated with rising living standards, an effective welfare state, regulation and so on—to which we can revert while saving the planet.

But whereas Daly's eco-friendly capitalism is 'small-scale' and stationary, under Pollin's 'green new deal', a bigger economy may be better. This is a key difference. Ironically, the name 'green new deal' was popularized by *New York Times* columnist and ardent free-marketeer Thomas Friedman in 2007.[13] Friedman is in favour of capitalist solutions to the climate crisis because he believes in the preternatural power of the market: 'There is only one thing as big as Mother Nature, and that is Father Greed—a.k.a., the market. I am a green capitalist. I think we will only get the scale we need by shaping the market.'[14] Pollin, on the

---

[13] Thomas Friedman, 'A Warning From the Garden', *New York Times*, 19 January 2007.
[14] Thomas Friedman, 'The Green New Deal Rises Again', *NYT*, 8 January 2019.

other hand, obviously no fan of 'Father Greed', and for whom 'green capitalist' is a flagrant misnomer, believes in the social value of healthy growth rates. This is his priority, and his sense of the urgency of the climate crisis means that while he does discuss how different owner-ship forms might advance his renewables agenda, he is prepared to postpone the question of an alternative economic order.

Why is growth such a priority for Pollin? That it is becomes particularly evident, paradoxically, when he is ostensibly conceding its deficiencies:

> It is obvious that growth *per se*, as an economic category, makes no refer-ence to the distribution of the costs and benefits of an expanding economy. As for Gross Domestic Product as a statistical construct, aiming to measure economic growth, there is no disputing that it fails to account for the pro-duction of environmental bads.

Unwilling to give up on growth itself, he distances it from what he calls variously 'growth *per se*', or growth 'as an economic category', or GDP 'as a statistical construct'. Though the paragraph begins with Pollin assur-ing us that he shares 'virtually all the values and concerns of degrowth advocates', by its end, one has the sense that all he has really conceded is that GDP is an imperfect measure because it fails to tell us a lot of important information about economies other than their size—a point with which Daly would of course agree. Pollin's wish to preserve growth by surrounding it with this thicket of qualifications is partly explained by the funding mechanism that underpins his programme: since invest-ment comes from a portion of global GDP, 'a higher economic-growth rate will also accelerate the rate at which clean energy supplants fossil fuels'.[15] But this is to beg the question, since one must then ask why Pollin decides to tie his programme's investment prospects to global growth rates. Although he does not dwell on them here, it becomes clear that there are two, connected reasons Pollin remains commit-ted to growth. Firstly, he regards it as politically non-negotiable: 'most political leaders remain convinced that significantly cutting fossil-fuel dependency will slow economic growth and cost jobs—a price they are

---

[15] Burton and Somerville reject this claim, arguing that Pollin ignores the fact that a faster-growing economy will be using more energy, thus annulling the progress made by a speedier transition: though moving faster up it, we will simply be adding 'to the hill that has to be climbed' by renewable-energy systems.

unwilling to pay.'[16] If this is the brute political fact from which all green strategizing must begin, as it is for Pollin, then the only meaningful path forward is to develop policy instruments that will allow politicians to oversee major losses to fossil-fuel industries while sustaining healthy growth rates overall.

But Pollin's commitment to growth is not simply pragmatic: author of *Back to Full Employment* (2012), he also recognizes that growth means jobs, and he believes that 'the single best form of protection' for workers in all countries who are displaced by the switch to clean energy—more than 'adjustment assistance programmes', like retraining and relocating workers—is 'a full-employment economy' in which 'there is an abundance of decent jobs available for all people seeking work'.[17] Correspondingly, Pollin's central objection to degrowth is to its 'immediate effect': 'huge job losses and declining living standards for working people and the poor'. This prospect is in turn a central reason that maintaining growth is politically compulsory. Pollin says he has 'not seen a convincing argument from a degrowth advocate' about how to avoid this eventuality. Can Burton and Somerville be said to supply one? They support Pollin's call for a 'just transition'—but who would oppose it?—and suggest that the rich world and high-income consumers would be hit hardest. But in the short term at least, the effects of their 'drastic' cuts in industrial food and goods production, construction and international trade would send prices soaring, while millions would be thrown out of work.

Displacement

Whatever the persuasiveness of its application to Pollin, Burton and Somerville's complaint of a 'misidentification of the villain(s)' helps explain why Kunkel's remark about GDP provoked such sustained response. One of the reasons for this ripple effect might be that it enabled a minor displacement of the argument.[18] For another faultline in the series—a line that recedes from the prominence one would expect of

---

[16] Pollin, 'Global Green Growth for Human Development', p. 3.
[17] Pollin, 'Global Green Growth for Human Development', p. 15.
[18] This is not to suggest that such 'displacement' is evasive, or leads to irrelevant quibbling: the discussion about the significance and durability of GDP is one of the liveliest threads of the debate.

it—separates those who envisage saving the world within the framework of a mitigated capitalism (Pollin, and, somewhat half-heartedly, Daly), from those who think averting climate catastrophe means ridding ourselves of the economic system largely responsible for it (Vettese, Burton and Somerville).

But though the difference this faultline marks is fundamental—one between political-economic systems that are not simply alternatives, but *incompatible* alternatives—it is not always immediately discernible. This is partly because contributors on both sides of the line—whether because they are unwilling or merely uninterested—mostly do not explicitly categorize their proposals in these terms. Daly doesn't think 'we should just abandon capitalism and opt for eco-socialism', yet he also says that if you want to call his more egalitarian brand of capitalism, 'eco-socialism, that's fine with me'.

The anti-capitalists are similarly casual about how to classify their policies politically. Like Daly, Vettese is pluralistic: 'The project might take on any number of mantles: "egalitarian eco-austerity", "eco-socialism" or, borrowing from Wilson, "half-earth economics".' That is the only time Vettese uses the word 'socialism'—its radical edge blunted by being enclosed in quotation marks and preceded by a prefix. And though Burton and Somerville speak of the 'collapse of the capitalist system', they also slightly hedge their mention of socialism with a qualification that makes it sound indeterminate or approximate: 'an ecologically sustainable world economy' would require 'a socialist mode of production of some sort'.

This evasion of binding political distinctions has visible consequences. Instead of debating whether the planetary rescue operation can be conducted within the capitalist system—or, if not, what would be required to establish a different economic order within which it could—much of the argument, spurred on by Kunkel's opening comment, becomes focused on growth, and its compatibility with ecological recovery. So part of the point of insisting, as Burton and Somerville do, that neoliberalism is continuous with mid-twentieth-century kinds of capitalism, and that both are equally beholden to the profit-making imperative, is to demonstrate that capitalism—including, necessarily, the ongoing economic expansion it requires—is, indeed, the villain. In other words, the crux of the disagreement is not exactly about the benefits of untrammelled growth—which no-one, including Pollin, is unequivocally in favour of—but about whether or not growth as such is ecologically destructive. If, like Daly, Burton and Somerville and other degrowth advocates, you think the answer to this question is 'yes', then the question becomes whether or not growth-limitation or shrinkage can happen with the basic parameters of the capitalist system still in place (Daly, yes; Burton and Somerville, probably not).

To revert to the question that was slightly dislodged by the discussion of GDP following Kunkel's contentious claim: is capitalism capable of ecological self-healing, or does it, as well as fossil-fuelled growth, need to be jettisoned if the planet is to remain habitable? Broadly speaking Daly and Pollin seem to converge in thinking capitalism can prevent the worst of the oncoming climate crisis—as long as it is prevented by massive state intervention from doing *its* worst. Of course, Daly and Pollin are not free-market ideologues but pragmatists who start from the conviction that capitalism is what we're stuck with for the moment, and we haven't got much time. They do not believe that markets will be the sole agent of the transition to clean energy. If they did, they would presumably have nothing to add to the debate, since the problem of 'what is to be done' would magically dissolve: we could simply sit back, relax and watch capitalism autopilot itself to ecological repair.

Vettese raises cautious reservations about capitalism's capacity to fix the crisis it partly precipitated: he believes that state-inflected market solutions to the climate crisis like those offered by Daly 'underestimate the difficulties of shackling capitalism so as to slow it down'. Taking the view that the industrial-scale contractions of the economy necessary to protect the planet are unlikely to take place within a mitigated capitalism that 'leaves the overall system of commodification, and the motors of expansion, firmly in place', Burton and Somerville possibly put it more strongly, suggesting that the necessary downsizing will probably happen only after some kind of breakdown of the prevailing economic order.

There are reasons to be doubtful about the idea that ridding the planet of capitalism is the answer to the ecological crisis we face. Firstly, though we must surely acknowledge the minimum fact that 'there is a link between capitalism and emissions of carbon dioxide', at least since the adoption of coal at the onset of industrialization, we must also ask whether the link between economic activity and ecological impact is distinctive of this mode of production.[19] Communism, too—famously, in both the Soviet and Chinese cases—has been no less devastating for the environment in recent times, if over a briefer historical period. The industrialization of the USSR and the PRC was not at all different, in ecological terms, from that of their capitalist counterparts with whom they were trying to catch up. 'All modern states', Michael Mann writes, 'have sacrificed the environment to GDP, regardless of regime type.' Indeed, Mann is convinced that 'if we all had state socialism, the problem would be just the same'. Perhaps this is partly why the contributors have mostly preferred to concentrate on the basic principle of cutting consumption, rather than on the finer details of who owns the means of production.

Instrumentalizing the crisis?

Mann identifies three 'fundamental social actors of our time' whom he thinks are responsible for climate change: capitalism, nation-states and individual consumers. For Mann, avoiding planetary disaster is a matter of curbing the powers of all three. He makes two other important points about the kind of problem climate change poses: it is 'a genuinely global issue'—'emissions in all countries affect everyone's climate' so 'legislation must be international', and—though the time-span in which meaningful action can be taken is getting shorter—it is a long-term problem.[20] These factors combine to make solving the climate crisis particularly difficult: short-termism characterizes the thinking of both politicians, beholden to the rhythm of election cycles, and the capitalist classes, bound to the profit-making imperative, whilst the nation-state remains the fundamental political and jurisdictional unit, and the performance of the national economy, the overriding political priority. These conditions encourage or compel governments to keep kicking the ecological can down the road. Everyone's problem and no one's problem, it is an international crisis that has not yet become any nation's domestic priority. Until and unless it does so, it seems clear that the necessary sacrifices will not be made.

Bearing in mind Mann's pointers about the specific difficulties climate change presents, can any conclusions be drawn from this comparative survey of the debate so far about the kind of strategizing that is required?

---

[19] Andreas Malm, 'Long Waves of Fossil Development: Periodizing Energy and Capital', *Mediations*, vol. 31, no. 2, Spring 2018, p. 17.
[20] Mann, *The Sources of Social Power*, pp. 366, 362, 380.

It seems unarguable that an essential component of any viable green strategy must be the existence of a global, intergovernmental body with genuine legislative capabilities and practical powers of implementation. The problem with Pollin's programme is that it assumes that this kind of truly effective international organization either already exists, or could easily be created. Recent UN climate talks suggest this assumption is unjustified. The central strategic question, then, is how to mobilize global green coalitions that would make such a transnational body genuinely cooperative, productive and powerful—which might require governments to accept severe limitations on their national sovereignty.[21]

Putting the question this way also provides an opportunity for a critique of capitalism—rather than just of growth—that goes beyond enumerating the ways in which it is a socially blighted and ecocidal system, or providing apophatic, counterfactual arguments about the environmental fringe benefits if capitalism were to be replaced with an alternative economic order. That means producing evidence to support the claim that capitalism is not only killing the planet, but that the geopolitical arrangements it enshrines are what is preventing us from taking necessary action to save it.

An example of this kind of argument is given in *Climate Leviathan*. There, Geoff Mann and Joel Wainwright argue that globalized capitalism is itself an impediment to cooperation on a world scale, since—though it gives rise to economic interdependence—it also heightens inter-state competitiveness and exacerbates global inequality, which 'undermines the capacity for collective action by reducing willingness to share sacrifices'.[22] This economic inequality is intensified by a kind of ecological inequality: the skewed geographical distribution of where ecological harm is predominantly caused, and where it is most felt. While Michael Mann is right to point out that 'carbon emissions anywhere affect everywhere' since 'the climate knows no boundaries', it is also true that these effects are uneven: rich, high-emitting citizens of the global North continue to bear most of the responsibility for the warming of the planet, while poorer citizens of the global South are most likely to suffer the unpredictable consequences. These low-emitting countries are also

---

[21] To increase 'the power of the collectivity of nation-states', it might be necessary to reduce their individual autonomy. See Mann, *The Sources of Social Power*, p. 380.
[22] Geoff Mann and Joel Wainwright, *Climate Leviathan: A Political Theory of Our Planetary Future*, London and New York 2018, p. 101.

less well-resourced when it comes to recovering from environmental calamities. It is the problem of how to overcome such economic and ecological unevenness—and how to compel high-consuming countries to accept sacrifices on behalf of the safety and sustainability of low-consuming countries—that is so intractable.

Vettese is alert to these issues: he discusses the way environmentalist programmes can 'ossify the inequality between the global North and South', since the former's development was enabled by an offloading of its ecological costs onto the latter, whose own, more recent development is now being regulated by the richer countries. Vettese claims that this 'hypocrisy has prevented greens from building coalitions across international borders and between social movements, but the half-earthing adoption of the 2,000-watt framework would overcome this history of division', since 'it would allow the poorest to double or triple their consumption, while requiring a commensurate reduction by the rich.' The difficulty here is that Vettese does not explain how this drastic reduction in consumption would be accomplished in advanced economies without the hemispheric divisions he identifies *already* being overcome—assuming, that is, that such radical policies would require the international green coalitions the current system prevents to already exist.

Moral and ecological arguments abound for consuming less and organizing our economies more thoughtfully and fairly, and in ways that show greater respect for nature, as well as each other (and these arguments are in plentiful supply in the series so far). But, as Mann writes, though 'eco-socialist arguments are morally valid, morality does not rule the world'—even if it does, as Daly and Kunkel discuss, have some 'material effect on how things happen'.[23] If Pollin's contribution disappoints because it doesn't articulate any broader socio-economic vision, more radical, composite contributions can encounter the opposite problem, which is that the concern for social and economic justice can seem to predominate over ecological considerations. These last can then come to seem tacked on or subsidiary. Rather than lining up arguments for why we need to combat capitalism and climate change in one fell swoop, eco-socialist visions can leave one with the impression that they are proposing to kill the two birds with one stone—instrumentalizing

---

[23] Mann, *The Sources of Social Power*, p. 390.

the climate crisis to co-opt its urgency in order to expedite socialist transformation.[24] However sympathetic one is to the latter aspiration, there is a danger that the result of this opportunism will be to drain the eco-socialist hybrid strategy of its political plausibility and to achieve nothing—neither its social nor its ecological objectives.

Given this, are there political projects which not only combine social and economic justice with ecological rescue, but integrate them so tightly that they become structurally dependent[25]—not just once the transition has already been made, and we are comfortably settled in our eco-socialist world, but prior to this hypothetical transition? It may be true that 'it is easier to imagine the end of the world than to imagine the end of capitalism',[26] but can it be shown that we need to attempt the latter—the hardly imaginable—in order to prevent the former—the easily imaginable— from befalling us in reality?

Pragmatic impossibilism vs utopian realism

Pollin's political pragmatism—his avoidance of radical restrictions and fairness measures, his exclusive focus on where we get our energy from, and his reticence about making evaluative or normative claims about how we ought to live—is, as we saw, what makes his proposal seem plausible. But is Pollin's variety of *Realpolitik* as pragmatic as it seems in the context of a crisis of such scale and urgency? Does pursuing the unimaginable or advocating the impossible paradoxically have a greater chance of effecting change at the magnitude and speed required? This is to pose a final, meta-strategic question about

---

[24] Listen, for example, to how Naomi Klein describes her awakening to environmentalism: 'I began to understand how climate change . . . could become a galvanizing force for humanity, leaving us all not just safer from extreme weather, but with societies that are safer and fairer in all kinds of other ways as well . . . This is a vision of the future that goes beyond just surviving or enduring climate change, beyond "mitigating" and "adapting" to it in the grim language of the United Nations. It is a vision in which we collectively use the crisis to leap somewhere that seems, frankly, better than where we are right now': *This Changes Everything*, p. 7. The instrumentalism—'use the crisis'—is here undisguised.
[25] See, for example, George Monbiot's 'scheme for tackling climate change', which aims to be 'fair and progressive' only because 'that is what would make it politically plausible . . . Let us hammer the rich by other means, but let us not confuse this programme with an attempt to cut carbon emissions': 'Environmental Feedback', p. 112.
[26] Fredric Jameson, 'Future City', NLR 21, May–June 2003.

the appropriate or expedient posture one should assume in climate change debates.

In 'Who Will Build the Ark?', a text that precedes this series but informs much of its discussion, Mike Davis stages his own psychological oscillations 'between analytic despair and utopian possibility'. Davis's conclusion in that text was that 'on the basis of the evidence before us, taking a "realist" view of the human prospect, like seeing Medusa's head, would simply turn us into stone.' It can be reasonable and prudent to make overambitious, unrealistic demands, as Davis explains: 'Only a return to explicitly utopian thinking can clarify the minimal conditions for the preservation of human solidarity in face of convergent planetary crises.' Davis's species of utopianism is judicious, for just because it is so drastic, it illuminates what is indispensable and essential: 'the minimal conditions' for human survival, 'the Necessary rather than the merely Practical'. Realism and utopianism are thus not always simple opposites: utopianism can be strategic, in some version of what Francis Mulhern, writing about *n+1* and referring to one of its founding editors, Mark Greif, calls 'calculated impossibilism'—in Greif's words, 'asking for what is at present impossible, in order to get at last, by indirection or implausible directness, the principles that would underlie the world we'd want rather than the one we have'.[27]

Yet, propelling Davis's lurches between hopelessness and utopianism is the perception that reality—the all too real prospect of global disaster—has become, so to speak, *unrealistic*. What is scientifically 'necessary' to avert this disaster may be politically 'impossible': 'Either we fight for "impossible" solutions to the increasingly entangled crises of urban poverty and climate change, or become ourselves complicit in a *de facto* triage of humanity.' The scare quotes provide some small hope that these solutions are not truly impossible, but only 'impossible', and that the humanitarian catastrophe is preventable as well as our complicity in it. Yet there is a sense that this hopefulness is bred by a despair of alternatives, and is a reflex response to the dread that the two realities—scientific and political—may not harmonize in time.[28]

During the latest dispiriting episode of the UN climate talks, held in Katowice in December, Wells Griffith, Trump's international energy and

---

[27] Francis Mulhern, 'A Party of Latecomers', NLR 93, May–June 2015, pp. 82–3.
[28] Mike Davis, 'Who Will Build the Ark?', NLR 61, Jan–Feb 2010.

climate adviser, insisted: 'We strongly believe that no country should have to sacrifice their economic prosperity or energy security in pursuit of environmental sustainability.'[29] Here is eloquent evidence for the truth of Jameson's claim about our imaginative capacities, only twisted to express preference: Wells Griffith would apparently rather die with the world than live to see the end of capitalism. Or rather, perhaps, the end of America.

For this is what a devotion to GDP also means: as an index of the size of *national* economies, it is not just a commitment to the economy over the environment, it is a commitment to the *nation* over the rest of the world—and not just to the national economy, but to national security.[30] Indeed, the former is the key to the latter, since economic strength is critical for the industrial militarization that helps ensure geopolitical dominance. And, to cite another of Michael Mann's terse formulae: 'The more militarized a country is, the more it damages the environment.' Among the ways, as Mann points out, of enhancing national security—'currently the most sacred goal of American politicians'—is to achieve 'resource independence', by, for example, seeking out new fossil-fuel reserves on home soil in order to reduce dependence on imported oil. The irony, then, is that what countries do in the name of 'national security' may help to imperil the ecological security of the planet they share.[31]

In the month before the Katowice talks, a US climate report warned—echoing the metaphysical absurdity of Griffith's putting the economy before the planet (as if the former could proceed without the continued existence of the latter)—that global warming could reduce America's GDP by 10 per cent by the end of the century.[32] Not confined to undoing decades of economic progress in developing (and comparatively ecologically innocent) countries, climate change is set to shrink the world's largest and most ecologically culpable economies, too. Based on this

---

[29] Editorial Board, 'Trump Imperils the Planet', *New York Times*, 26 December 2018.
[30] J. R. McNeill thinks that 'among the swirl of ideas, policies and political structures of the twentieth century, the most ecologically influential probably were the growth imperative and the (not unrelated) security anxiety that together dominated policy around the world': *Something New Under the Sun*, p. 355.
[31] Mann, *The Sources of Social Power*, pp. 365, 376.
[32] Coral Davenport and Kendra Pierre-Louis, 'US Climate Report Warns of Damaged Environment and Shrinking Economy', *New York Times*, 23 November 2018.

report—leaving aside the distressing implications of its inhuman economism (one can imagine a scenario where it makes 'economic sense' to allow much of the planet, including many of its inhabitants, to go to waste)[33]—if the developed world doesn't degrow now, by choice, it will be degrown later, by force. The logic of the warning—save the planet to save (America's) GDP—suggests that if 'fidelity to GDP amounts to the religion of the modern world', the faith of the modern world's leading per capita polluter shows no sign of waning. Yet it also implies that even if the rich world's GDP idols are not to be smashed, the ecological gods may still punish its devotion to them.

---

[33] See Monbiot's critique of such attempts to calculate the 'economics of climate change' in 'Environmental Feedback', pp. 109–11.

Read.
Debate.
Organise.

Join the Left Book Club

A subscription book club for everyone on the left.

Mass membership of the LBC in the 1930s and 40s helped to turn public opinion against fascism and bring about Labour's landslide victory after WWII.

Join us today. You will receive:

• The best books from a range of publishers on politics, economics, society and culture
• Beautiful collectable editions, unique to members
• Choice of subscriptions at affordable prices
• Access to reading groups and events
• Build networks and champion political education

 Become a member:
www.leftbookclub.com

REVIEWS

Francis Mulhern, *Figures of Catastrophe: The Condition of Culture Novel*
Verso: London and New York 2016, £16.99, hardback
165 pp, 978 1 78478 191 0

FREDERIK VAN DAM

FICTIONS OF CULTURE

In one of Matthew Arnold's most celebrated lyrics, 'Dover Beach', the
speaker projects his state of mind onto the sea, which he perceives as cold,
unfeeling and foreign. Only at the beginning of the fourth stanza does he
find some kind of comfort, in the presence of a beloved. But even this brief
glimpse of hope is undercut and quickly gives way to disenchantment:

> Ah, love, let us be true
> To one another! For the world, which seems
> To lie before us like a land of dreams,
> So various, so beautiful, so new,
> Hath really neither joy, nor love, nor light,
> Nor certitude, nor peace, nor help for pain;
> And we are here as on a darkling plain
> Swept with confused alarms of struggle and flight,
> Where ignorant armies clash by night.

'Dover Beach' appeared in Arnold's last collection of poetry, *New Poems*
(1867), which was a swan-song of sorts: Arnold seems to have felt that
poetry was unable to alter human conduct in ways appropriate to modern
life. He therefore turned to criticism, in an attempt to craft the conditions
that would reinvigorate poetry's potential to do so. One of his most significant contributions to criticism was, in his preface to *Culture and Anarchy*
(1869), the redefinition of culture as 'a pursuit of our total perfection by

means of getting to know, on all the matters which most concern us, the best which has been thought and said in the world, and, through this knowledge, turning a stream of fresh and free thought upon our stock notions and habits'. It was through the cultivation of this disposition that men of different classes would be able to meet on equal terms. Shedding light on the darkling plain of the present, culture would abolish the typically English religion of inequality. Born out of his experiences on the Continent, this definition of culture was a controversial one, as it challenged an older and very different idea of culture as a set of customs and traditions: given the weight that patriotism carried in Victorian public discourse, many of Arnold's fellow citizens would have been reluctant to alienate themselves from this more traditional notion. As a result, the Arnoldian quest for culture became something of a phantom formation, its potential unrealized and its purposiveness elusive. It is this constitutive instability that gave rise to a discourse in which culture began to speak about itself and its conditions of existence.

In an earlier study, *Culture/Metaculture* (2000), Francis Mulhern charted the course of this discourse in the twentieth century while, from the sidelines, taking aim at many of its practitioners for collapsing the sphere of politics into that of aesthetics. Statements in metacultural discourse, in Mulhern's analysis, tend to usurp the place of judgements that properly belong to the domain of politics. It is this observation that led Mulhern to posit a hidden continuity between the elitist cultural criticism of the first half of the twentieth century (as practised by such different figures as F. R. Leavis and T. S. Eliot) and the more popular criticism within the discipline of Cultural Studies of the second half (whose foundational figure is Stuart Hall). Mulhern's characterization of these two seemingly opposite schools of thought and the implication that they are antagonistic variants of a shared metacultural discourse did not go unchallenged, however. In the pages of this journal, for instance, Stefan Collini's review sparked a critical exchange. It was from this 'timely provocation', as Mulhern describes it, that his new book was born. In *Figures of Catastrophe*, Mulhern examines how metacultural discourse sustains a current in the twentieth-century novel: not only do these novels suggest the usurpation of the place of politics in metacultural discourse, but they arguably do so in the name of a specific selectivity—the 'best that has been thought and said'—within the totality of significations that comprise any given culture. Mulhern thus effectively taxes what he calls the 'condition of culture' novel with performing a double distortion, masking an order of power as an order of meanings, and doing so in the name of a particular, arbitrary hierarchy of meanings.

One of the fundamental insights of *Figures of Catastrophe* is the observation that the matter of culture has been dealt with in novels, presumably that most bourgeois of literary forms. For Arnold, after all, it was only in (classical) poetry that an imaginative engagement with the conditions of modernity could be staged. Many later thinkers about culture also favoured the lyric. W. B. Yeats famously lamented that in the present 'all neglect / monuments of unaging intellect'. T. S. Eliot, too, clothed his critical metier with his authority as a poet. And in 'Cultural Criticism and Society', Theodor Adorno declaimed that 'to write poetry after Auschwitz is barbaric'. To suggest that the novel has taken part in the development of metacultural discourse is thus not self-evident. Perhaps this built-in lack of affinity partly explains why, as Mulhern shows, the twentieth-century novel proved to be an inhospitable environment for Arnold's critical enterprise.

Mulhern raises the stakes by suggesting that these metacultural novels constitute a distinctive genre—the 'condition of culture' novel. He maintains that it has its roots in the industrial novel, a nineteenth-century form in which a widespread social problem is dramatized through its effect on characters of flesh and blood. In the more modern genre of the condition of culture novel, this social problem takes shape as the threat posed to culture by, to stick with Arnold's critical vocabulary, various forms of anarchy, or, to use Mulhern's term, figures of catastrophe. In his definition of the genre, Mulhern opts for a flexible framework, which allows him to draw very different texts into his ken. In his introduction, he conceptualizes genre 'in the broad traditions of Georg Lukács and Mikhail Bakhtin' as applying 'at a relatively low level of historical generality, identifying groups of texts sharing a distinctive topic or set of topics'. Although these criteria are strongly thematic and may seem quite arbitrary at first (next to *Bildung*, 'topics' include suburbanization and the consumer economy), Mulhern's readings illustrate that these very different novels chime in with one another, often in unexpected and illuminating ways. His selection also has the benefit of overriding the distinction between modernism and post-modernism, thus yielding a more comprehensible picture of twentieth-century fiction than studies which insist on these two shibboleths.

In the readings that follow, Mulhern frequently has recourse to a particular method. Inspired by Fredric Jameson, he creatively reshapes Algirdas Julien Greimas's figure of the semiotic square. As Mulhern points out, the square often adds little to what is not already apparent in other ways, but it can be a powerful interpretative aid and reveal narrative possibilities that are not always visible to the naked eye. In Virginia Woolf's *Orlando*, for instance, Mulhern detects a non-necessary opposition between 'nobility' and 'literature', which has 'reputation' as its narrative resolution. This in turn produces a second opposition between 'common people' (the non-resolvable opposition of 'nobility') and 'life' (opposed to 'literature'), which has 'obscurity' as its narrative resolution. The newly formed opposition between 'nobility' and 'life' creates another outcome, 'ecstasy', whereas that between 'literature' and 'common people' creates 'calm'. The peculiarity of this particular square is that all the narrative resolutions ('reputation', 'obscurity', 'ecstasy', 'calm') are present in the novel and all of them put the protagonist, Orlando, in a favourable position. The novel thus creates 'an unchallengeable ideal of cultural wholeness'. As Mulhern concludes, Orlando's development 'is not the outcome of transforming contact with others—as in Margaret's case in *Howards End*, for example—but rather a process of self-elaboration'. In short, the semiotic square reveals how in *Orlando* the Arnoldian ideal of culture has become deeply narcissistic.

Arnold's significance for the history of the condition of culture novel comes to the fore most visibly in Mulhern's first chapter, in which he points out how the drama of E. M. Forster's *Howards End* is coded in the terms of Arnold's tribute to Sophocles, 'who saw life steadily and saw it whole'. In Mulhern's reading, *Howards End* suggests that the attempt to reinvigorate bourgeois liberalism with working-class aspiration takes a toll on the latter, personified by Leonard Bast. Through his association with the Schlegels, Bast is not completely alone in his quest for culture: *Howards End* anticipates a moment when men and women will be made equal by their common humanity, even though Bast will not live to see it. In Thomas Hardy's *Jude the Obscure*, in contrast, the perfunctory utopianism of *Howards End* is wholly absent: its working-class protagonist, Jude Fawley, is continually and tragically thwarted. By pairing these two novels, Mulhern highlights their shared sympathy for the victims of ruling-class arrogance, even if they fail to represent a convincing alternative. Later novelists are less keen to extend such sympathy, as he shows in the next three chapters.

The book's second chapter, 'The Aristocratic Fix', focuses on the interbellum. Mulhern suggests that Woolf's *Orlando* and *Between the Acts* explore two complementary narrative trajectories: whereas in *Orlando* the aristocracy is figured as the guarantor of cultural continuity, in *Between the Acts* the opposite holds true, with what passes for culture slowly dissolving into petty-bourgeois sociability. These two different trajectories are combined, so Mulhern argues, in Evelyn Waugh's *Brideshead Revisited*, a connection that is as surprising as it is revealing: although Woolf's secular worldview chafes against Waugh's Augustinian pessimism, Mulhern deftly shows how these two writers meet when it comes to the matter of culture. Both believe culture to be under threat, even as they locate the origin of this threat in different places: for Woolf it is the entrepreneurial middlebrow, while for Waugh it is the philistine plebeian. The narratives from the post-war era that Mulhern explores in his third chapter, 'The Horror . . .', further showcase characters who are not qualified for the knowledge that culture is supposed to offer, and who threaten the existence of those who are. In Elizabeth Bowen's *The Heat of the Day*, Stan Barstow's *A Kind of Loving*, John

REVIEWS

Fowles's *The Collector* and Ruth Rendell's *A Judgement in Stone,* the 'horror' that Mulhern's title refers to appears in the guise of militant socialism or the outgrowths of the welfare state. The final chapter, 'End-States', spans the period from the 1980s to the present day. Martin Amis's *Money,* V. S. Naipaul's *The Enigma of Arrival* and *The Mimic Men,* Hanif Kureishi's *The Black Album* and Zadie Smith's *On Beauty* suggest, in different ways, that the enabling conditions of culture have disintegrated through the pressure exerted by the cocktail of neo-liberal capitalism and colonialism.

The most substantial part of *Figures of Catastrophe* is its concluding essay, in which Mulhern picks out common themes, such as the significance of books and houses, while also drawing distinctions between, for instance, narratives of situation and narratives of transformation. His observations are persuasive; if the previous chapters are often linked through association, here he provides a more rigorous picture in which the individual parts are made to reappear with flair and sophistication. It therefore feels churlish to summarize two missed opportunities that Mulhern himself identifies. As he points out, this is a decidedly Anglo-Saxon history of the genre, which would gain much from a comparative perspective. He provides some helpful suggestions about the development of the condition of culture novel in the United States and Germany, but even here his vantage-point remains distinctly UK-centric: while he points out that the English genre is marked by the specificity of the class struggle, he is less clear about what might distinguish other variants. This omission is striking: in Germany especially, the decline of culture cannot be understood without reference to National Socialism, which was a very different kind of catastrophe.

Another reservation one might voice is that Mulhern's focus on class issues tends to obfuscate the importance of gender. To be sure, he demonstrates that in these novels the search for culture is decidedly masculine, and briefly pauses to reflect on the ways the female characters may 'embody' culture, or function as obstacles to it. But there is more to be said. Even though most of the prominent figures in metacultural discourse and metacultural fiction have been men, one must also recognize that culture has a long-standing association with the feminine, up until the present day. One of Arnold's main efforts, in fact, was his attempt at rescuing 'sweetness and light' from the feminization that it had received from the likes of John Ruskin. Mulhern does not linger on this paradox, but it is to his credit that he has created a framework for future investigations into the gendered aspects of metacultural discourse, be it in the novel or academic criticism.

In a more positive way, *Figures of Catastrophe* provides a fresh and innovative contribution to the study of the politics of intertextuality, which will be of interest to scholars working in reception history. One way in which cultural discourse reflects on its own conditions of possibility, Mulhern contends, is through the practice of citation. 'Dover Beach' affords an instance of this practice: as Isobel Armstrong puts it in *Victorian Poetry* (1993), the poem's final scene 'recalls a crucial text for Oxford intellectuals, Thucydides's account of the battle of Epipolae, a night battle in which the Athenians, not being able to tell friend from foe, fought one another'. Mulhern shows in great detail how the condition of culture novel, too, uses allusions and paraphrases to establish within the novel an image of what competences the reader should possess. He pays careful attention to the difference between the way in which the process of cultural evaluation is acted out in the narrated world of the novel and the way in which the discourse of culture appears, at a higher level, in 'the distribution of cultural capital' between writer and reader. In a cunning manner, Mulhern plays a similar game with his own readers. For instance, discussing how Forster in *Howards End* examined the fact that his liberal culture depended on 'an illiberal entrepreneurial class fraction that it conventionally disdained' as well as 'a labouring population to which it extended little more than disquieted solicitude', Mulhern sums up as follows: 'after such knowledge, what resolution?' Readers familiar with T. S. Eliot's poetry will recognize that Mulhern alludes to a line from 'Gerontion'—'After such knowledge, what forgiveness?' Even though Eliot plays only a minor part in this book, this reference suggests that his influence cannot be circumvented.

Perhaps one might go further and consider Mulhern's allusion as an actualization, from a critical rather than a post-colonial point of view, of the kind of mimicry that he so deftly analyses in the novels of V. S. Naipaul. A similar act of appropriation is evident in the chapter title, 'The Horror . . .' The allusion to Kurtz's dying words in Joseph Conrad's *Heart of Darkness* is tantalizing: does Mulhern mean to suggest that this novel's brutalization of Africans is somehow a prelude to the depiction of the figures of catastrophe in the post-war years? While these two instances may give the impression that *Figures of Catastrophe* is haunted by the conservative discourse that it analyses, one might also argue that Mulhern turns this discourse against itself. The second reading is strengthened by the fact that he often goes out of his way to take the reader by the hand, as when he translates the logical fallacy 'post hoc, ergo propter hoc' in a footnote. By thus playing with his readers' cultural competences, Mulhern 'performs' his thesis in his own criticism: his readers are made to feel, like characters in the condition of culture novel, that 'culture is its own cruelly satirical reward, dangerous at worst, and in all not worth the candle'.

Because of its close relation to *Culture/Metaculture*, *Figures of Catastrophe* will come in for scrutiny from certain corners. Just as Stefan Collini voiced reservations about the way in which Mulhern constructed the tradition of metacultural discourse, so I am not wholly convinced that the selection made here is representative of the many ways in which this discourse has been encoded in the modern novel. By defining culture in Raymond Williams's terms, and by positing that the condition of culture novel is a continuation of the industrial novel, Mulhern rules out the possibility that instead of being a social problem, culture might also be a platform for the promotion of equality. What if Mulhern had taken George Eliot's *The Mill on the Floss* instead of *Howards End* and *Jude the Obscure* as his beginning or—to enlist a more provocative candidate—Anthony Trollope's *Ayala's Angel*? Both, I think, meet Mulhern's requirement of being 'synoptic and specific, foregrounding the cultural dimension of the social whole, undertaking a synoptic narrative evaluation of the social relations of culture'. And what if Mulhern had chosen novels which highlight different modes or which can be decoded in different ways? Mulhern briefly considers the example of the *Bildungsroman* as an instance of a genre whose defining topic 'is everywhere in modern culture, far exceeding the recognizable boundaries of the genre proper'. Given that for Arnold, 'culture' was a cipher for *Bildung*, the *Bildungsroman* would have been an equally interesting model. From the beginning of the nineteenth century, English novelists have adapted the genre of the vocational novel to the context of a Britain in the throes of global capitalism. While Mulhern shows that the condition of culture novel is a creature of many hues, extending the range of his readings to include different, but equally well-qualified novels might have yielded a more complex picture.

If the seemingly self-evident way in which Mulhern assembles his corpus serves to hide potential fissures, the at first sight flexible theoretical framework also yields a number of questions. On the one hand, the book wears its theory lightly. Mulhern prefers to put concepts into practice rather than to elaborate them in detail. The fact that Greimas and Jameson are relegated to an extensive footnote is an instance of Mulhern's methodology. It is to be hoped that this hands-on approach will allow the study to reach the wide readership it deserves. On the other hand, the study would have been strengthened by a more elaborate justification of its theoretical premises. In particular, I think that to combine the Marxist ideas of Lukács with the formalist views of Bakhtin requires a more thorough explanation than Mulhern offers. He apparently takes his cue from Lukács's later work, such as *The Historical Novel*, in which Lukács examines how the genre entered a period of decline after the revolutions of 1848, when bourgeois novelists retreated from their ambition to express popular consciousness. Mulhern's narrative runs in a parallel fashion, insofar as he sees the condition of culture novel as a modified resumption of its prototype, the industrial novel. Bakhtin has a very different idea about the ideological uses to which the novel can be put: if for the later Lukács it reflects the ideological interests out of which it was born, for Bakhtin the form retains the potential to be subversive because it comes into being through the polyphonic play of different voices or discourses. While the idea of polyphony often crops up in Mulhern's argument, as when he writes that *Between the Acts* 'quickly establishes an imagery of natural violence that will persist as the novel's interpretive ground-bass', this idea often does not lead to the kind of complementary reading that the presence of Bakhtin in the introduction hints at, and which some of the novels that Mulhern selects lend themselves to. Indeed, some novels also tell a story about culture's emancipatory potential, and not just one of authoritarian exclusion. Take, for instance, *Brideshead Revisited*, in which one may fruitfully see a case of queer tutelage in the homosocial bond between Charles Ryder and Sebastian Flyte, who teaches Charles to see life as an art and whose aid leads to Charles's first commissions. At the centre of the novel, then, we find a moment in which characters manage to create the communal form of coexistence that, as Mulhern rightly points out, is cancelled out by the novel's melancholic conclusion, in which the ancient house becomes a garrison for soldiers who are unaware of its complex history. The novel thus has a part that resonates strongly with Mulhern's own findings even as it challenges some of his conclusions. It might have strengthened Mulhern's argument to acknowledge that the novel articulates a number of intellectual positions. Such an acknowledgement would also have given his salute to Bakhtin a stronger justification.

Mulhern's reference to the theories of Lukács is less problematic, but here, too, a difference should be noted. Like Lukács, Mulhern situates various novels in their respective periods, though without literally ascribing a given novel to a given mode of production. But Lukács also explicitly delivers aesthetic judgements on specific novels, explaining their strengths and weaknesses as works of art. Mulhern's judgement is tacit and essentially political rather than aesthetic. Given that the literary merits of some of the works in his canon are debatable, some assessment of them in terms of their successes and failings as aesthetic objects might have enhanced his detailed account of how they participate in the genre.

It is worth emphasizing this withholding of evaluative judgements, given murmurs of a return to a more properly 'critical' attitude in literary studies. I here use 'critical' in a specific sense, as Joseph North defines it in *Literary Criticism: A Concise Political History* (2017). According to North, literary criticism, properly understood, disappeared from the academic scene at some point during the late 1970s or early 1980s, when it was replaced with a variety of historicist and contextualist approaches. This turn to scholarship is often understood as a political victory for the liberal left: Fredric Jameson's muchheeded call to 'always historicize' helped to place Marxism at the centre of the discipline. But with this transformation of literary studies into social theory, the evaluative impulse behind literary criticism was lost, along with its ability to cultivate the aesthetic capabilities of readers. The left's victory, then, was Pyrrhic: the historicist attention to specific details came at the cost of isolating literary studies from the real world.

Given Mulhern's own interest in this turn, as his review of North's book in NLR 110 attests, it is noteworthy that *Figures of Catastrophe* seems closer to the scholarly than the critical end of the spectrum. The study's primary aim is contextualist in nature, as it essentially traces a social-political trajectory across twentieth-century Britain, into which each novel finds its place. However, Mulhern does not use this historicizing approach as the platform for a political manifesto. One could interpret Mulhern's conclusion that the condition of culture genre is a regressive form—there are few consolations in these novels for those who still believe in the redemptive and civilizing power of art—as a call for a progressive kind of literature that would alter human conduct and serve the interests of equality. But Mulhern is content to leave this interpretation up to the reader. This is arguably a wise choice: to deliver a political judgement would be to fall into the trap of metacultural discourse with which the condition of culture novel is affiliated and in which the aesthetic is effaced by the political. Mulhern might, however, have shed his tactical reserve and combined his historical account of the genre with a more evaluative diagnosis of individual works. The issue of the critic's personal taste is particularly relevant in a study that deals with genre, after all. For a critic such as John Frow (*Genre*, 2015), 'genre is not a property of a text but is a function of reading'. In his view, all readers have a cultural repertoire that functions as a filter for their reading of new texts—texts that will, in turn, create new or refined filters. Some of Mulhern's readers may want to use the condition of culture genre that he identifies as a filter to re-read works that might be illuminated by it, even if, in Mulhern's view, these novels do not fit the bill. Mulhern shows himself to be well-attuned to the different modes within the condition of culture novel, but is nevertheless quite authoritative in dividing the goats from the sheep.

Let me illustrate this final point by providing a more critical reading of a text that confirms the validity of Mulhern's theory even if it is one that Mulhern himself might not classify as a condition of culture novel. Ian McEwan's *Saturday* (2005), often designated as a post-9/11 novel, meets a number of the touchstones of the condition of culture novel, as in its circular movement, its autobiographical tone, and its concern with class, nationhood and family. Like many characters in contemporary condition of culture novels, McEwan's protagonist, Henry Perowne, is unreceptive to the civilizing power of culture. His daughter Daisy, a poet, has forced him to read *Madame Bovary* and *Anna Karenina*, which leave him unmoved. The novel's story illustrates how this dismissive attitude is perilous. Early in the day, Perowne's car collides with that of Baxter, a lower-class thug, on a London street that has been barricaded to control a sea of anti-war protesters. Perowne, a neurosurgeon, manages to escape unharmed by explaining that Baxter is suffering from Huntington's disease, thus defusing his aggression. Seeking revenge for this humiliating encounter, Baxter and a companion later invade Perowne's house and threaten to violate his daughter. She saves herself and her family by reciting 'Dover Beach', which both Baxter and Perowne mistake for her own work: overcome with emotion, Baxter drops his knife and asks Perowne for help. In this resolution, the signature of the condition of culture novel is clear. Daisy Perowne is a latter-day Miranda Grey, who uses her cultural resources to try and tame the latter-day Fred Clegg who has subdued her, while the novel's citation of Arnold's words is reminiscent of Forster's allusions in *Howards End*.

But is McEwan's portrait convincing? 'Are we really to believe', as John Banville wonders, 'that an intelligent and attentive man such as Henry Perowne, no matter how keen his scientific bent, would have passed through the English education system without ever having heard of Matthew Arnold?' Is Perowne's act of disinterestedness in saving Baxter's life consistent with his character, given that throughout the novel he has been pondering his own inability to control his destiny in a world of unsurpassed complexity? By reducing events like the war in Iraq to occasions for self-regarding introspection, *Saturday* should be faulted for causing its readers to mistake the pleasures of melancholy introspection for heroic action. If literary criticism is to prompt readers to see culture as an inducement to commit oneself to real, material change, pregnant questions and fighting words such as these may be necessary. Of course, this attempt at a more evaluative stance and at moving beyond the strict limitations of the genre is only possible thanks to Mulhern's own thinking about the subject. I can only hope that it shows how *Figures of Catastrophe*, as a timely intervention on an important subject, is certain to stimulate further debate on the direction that literary criticism should take.

Stephen Smith, *La ruée vers l'Europe: La jeune Afrique en route pour le Vieux Continent*
Éditions Grasset & Fasquelle: Paris 2018, €19.50, paperback
272 pp, 978 2 24680 350 8

ALEXANDRA REZA

IMAGINED TRANSMIGRATIONS

Stephen Smith's *La ruée vers l'Europe* caused a ruckus when it appeared in France last year and the English translation, due out shortly from Polity under the title *The Scramble for Europe*, will no doubt have the same effect on this side of the Channel. A short book evidently aimed at a wide readership, *La ruée* extrapolates from present trends in African population growth and economic development to predict a large-scale rise in migration to Europe. Over the next two generations, Smith argues, 'more than 100 million Africans are likely to cross the Mediterranean Sea'; by 2050, 'between a fifth and a quarter of the European population would therefore be of African descent.' Some EU politicians, Smith writes, have hailed this as a 'demographic boon', Young Africa providing Old Europe with youth and diversity, 'brains and brawn'. In Smith's view, however, it would be a bad thing for both continents.

La ruée vers l'Europe was duly lauded by Emmanuel Macron, who told TV viewers that Smith had really hit the nail on the head and described the situation 'fantastically well'. His Foreign Minister, Jean-Yves Le Drian, hailed Smith's 'realist' diagnostic of the 'migrant crisis' and awarded the book a prize, as did the Académie française and *La Revue des deux mondes*. Meanwhile in *Le Monde diplomatique* Benoît Bréville characterized Smith's predictions as 'myths', arguing that the idea of a rush for Europe was a political fabrication. In *La Vie des idées*, the geographer Julien Brachet went further: 'Let's be clear: Smith's proposition is ideological, xenophobic and racist.' At face value, however, Smith's credentials don't suggest a hardened bigot. Born in Connecticut, educated in Paris and Berlin, a roving correspondent and then, for fifteen years, the Africa editor at *Libération*, Smith is perhaps best known in the Anglosphere for his contributions to the *London Review of Books* and plays a leading role in African and African-American Studies at Duke University. What is his case in *La ruée*, and how should it be evaluated?

Contrary to Macron and Le Drian's claims, Smith's book is not a description of existing reality—migration from Africa to Europe is low and falling; most African migration is within the continent—but a future projection, based on extrapolated population trends. Smith opens with the *longue durée* history of Africa, seen in demographic terms. Between 1500 and 1900, Smith estimates, the number of the continent's inhabitants rose by only 20 per cent, from 80 to 95 million, while populations quintupled in China and Europe. In 1650, Africans had made up a fifth of the world's population. By 1930 they counted for only 13 per cent. The explanation lay, first, with the slave trade, which involved the deportation of 28 million Africans by 1900, 12 million of those going to the Americas. Still more catastrophic was the microbial impact of nineteenth-century colonization, when between a third and a half of the people of West and Central Africa died from their encounter with imported diseases, at levels comparable to Europe's fourteenth-century Black Death.

One result was that, as *La ruée* puts it, the continent's population became its most valuable public good: while farming land was abundant, labour was precious. 'Wealth in people', socially and culturally structured through lineage groups, with a concomitant emphasis on inter-personal relations, became a driving force of African history, Smith argues. He cites *Facing Mount Kenya*, Kenyatta's memoir of life in a Kikuyu village around 1900. Kenyatta describes a society in which 'the homestead is the school', and where education centred on personal relationships and proper codes of conduct. Children learned through imitation of their elders, 'a rehearsal of the activities which are the serious business of all the members of the tribe'. The main objective was 'the building of character': for 'character is formed primarily through relations with other people, and there is really no other way in which it can grow. Europeans assume that, given the right knowledge and ideas, personal relations could take care of themselves.' This, Kenyatta thought, was 'the most fundamental difference in outlook' between Africans and Europeans.

On Smith's account, African population growth only began to recover in the interwar period but since then has accelerated 'at a rate never before seen in human history', as falling infant mortality rates have combined with low prevalence of modern contraception—below 15 per cent, *La ruée* notes—and a young average age of mothers at first birth. From 300 million in 1960, Sub-Saharan Africa's population had grown to a billion in 2010, and Smith projects a further rise to 2.5 billion by 2050 and to 5 billion by 2100, when on his estimate Africans will constitute 40 per cent of humanity. Already, he argues, this growth has had far-reaching socio-economic effects. First, while the continent is still predominantly rural—in the first decade of the twenty-first century, only 35 per cent of Africans lived in cities—there has been insufficient economic development in the countryside or at village level to accommodate the growing numbers of young people. According to Smith, 96 per cent of peasant farmers cultivate plots of less than 5 hectares, and cereal yield stands at 1.4 tons per hectare, compared to 8.1 tons in the US. Some 400 million still suffer from chronic malnutrition, which impairs the growth of 60 per cent of children. Accordingly, over the last few generations hundreds of millions of young Africans have left their villages, searching for work. But local towns and cities cannot absorb their labour either: 'Although they are themselves industrious, they have moved into cities with no industry, where they manage their lives, such as they are, on a day-to-day basis.' The next stage is the move from provincial town to regional hub: Abidjan, Lagos, Nairobi, Johannesburg. The continent's urban conglomerations have been growing at an even faster rate than its population: Dakar, Nairobi and Harare are all ten times bigger than they were in 1960; Khartoum and Mogadishu, twenty times; Kampala, Kinshasa and Ouagadougou, thirty times; Abidjan forty times and Lagos sixty times greater. By 2050, Smith estimates, 60 per cent of Africans will be living in large cities.

A second outcome of this population growth has been a revolutionary transformation in the ratio of young people to old: 80 per cent of the African population is now under 30. Given 'traditional' principles of seniority and 'respect for elders', Smith argues, this has had profound political and cultural effects. African governments are, by and large, 'gerontocracies', with an average age gap between rulers and ruled of 43 years, compared to 32 years in Latin America, 30 years in Asia and 16 years in the EU, with its ageing population. This discrepancy risks reducing young Africans to second-tier citizens, young women even more so. 'Cynically speaking', Smith writes, 'the value of human life has declined in inverse proportion to the continent's unprecedented population growth.' (This is indeed a profoundly cynical statement, and baffling too: there is no reason why quantitative increase in population need qualitatively devalue human life.) The treasuring of inter-personal relations that Kenyatta recalled is over, Smith implies. 'The price of what is available in abundance depreciates, while scarcity increases value. That rule applies today for young people in a world predominantly populated by older adults.' Citing Paul Collier, the English developmental economist best known for telling Africans to pick themselves up by their bootstraps, Smith argues that the 'youth bulge' endangers the continent's democratic future. Since huge proportions of the population in many Sub-Saharan countries are below the legal voting age, the ballot appears 'more an age-based privilege than a majoritarian right'. As such, Africa's youth 'destabilize democracy'.

Rebellion against the 'primacy of the elders' finds an ideological home in the new forms of religiosity that have swept the continent, Smith writes. He quotes from Nicolas Argenti's study of youth in Cameroon, which contends that Pentecostalism functions as a rejection of 'everything the elders stood for, effecting a continuous state of rupture with the past by means of continuous personal renewal, to establish a life free from enslavement by Satan—where Satan can be seen as an embodiment of the gerontocratic structures that so alienate the young.' Most significantly, for Smith, evangelical gospels of prosperity may presuppose a Protestant nuclear-family ethic that upends traditional rules of reciprocity and kinship ties, with born-again believers refusing to take in relatives or accusing them of 'sponging'—a radical break with previous norms. Smith notes that militant Islam in the Sahel region has sometimes mobilized as a revolutionary assault against ageing rulers' corruption.

Third, the frustrations of Africa's youth are being buoyed up on a shallow but real influx of prosperity. After two decades of stagnation, and lifted by China's drive for raw materials, African economies have finally 'reaped the dividends' of the painful structural-adjustment programmes imposed by the IMF in the 1980s, Smith declares. He deploys the familiar imagery of Rising Africa—skyscrapers and mud huts, 4G networks and talking drums. 'A new land of opportunities is rising out of an ocean of misery', and with it a new middle class, an estimated 130 million consumers, earning between $5 and $20 a day, who can therefore envisage meeting the costs of migration, around $2,500. In addition, these layers are increasingly online, saving up for mobile phones or using the ubiquitous digital kiosks. Smith suggests that the internet makes the dream worlds of American culture available at a click.

These are the conditions, La ruée argues, whose convergence around 2050 could produce the 'scramble for Europe' his book predicts. A continuous acceleration of population growth; rising strata whose progress has been blocked at home, yet who can look beyond their own country to imagine a new life in a far-away place and—'the sine qua non'—possess the financial means to undertake the journey. Although these factors have yet to materialize on the scale he foresees, in Smith's view they possess a 'numerical logic'. Once a certain tipping point is reached, 'internal migration within the continent will no longer function as an escape valve, and a large number of Africans will begin to push open the doors to the entire world, beginning with Europe.' The outcome is *inscrit dans l'ordre des choses*—written in the order of things.

This putative future sets the scene for *La ruée*'s discussion of how Europe should 'react'. Should Africans be allowed to enter in large numbers? Stopped at the borders? Filtered and 'profiled'? Smith explains he takes it 'as a given' that 'the host is an entitled figure on home turf'—otherwise, concepts of sovereignty and nation would no longer mean anything. Bearing that in mind, he comes up with five 'plausible scenarios' from which the citizens of Europe are invited to choose. The first, 'Eurafrica', envisages an Americanization of EU attitudes, welcoming the huddled masses from the south who will give the 'Old World' a younger, more diverse and dynamic population, along the lines of the 'welcome culture' extended by Germany in 2015. This scenario, Smith tells us, would be the 'triumph of a humanistic universalism', but if it were sustained, it would also require cutting back the social state to American levels. The second scenario is 'Fortress Europe': securing the borders. The advantage would be that genuine asylum-seekers would no longer have to compete with economic migrants, as Smith thinks happens presently. The disadvantage: though the borders could be tightened, as in 2017, it's illusory to think the coming 'scramble' could be stemmed by security measures alone.

'Mafia Drift' is the third scenario, somewhat vaguely envisaged: human traffickers, understood as not just enablers but causal factors in migration—selling the dream of a new life like so many drug dealers—could join forces with organized crime, or start a war against it, were the European underworld to find a far-right political patron. Fourth, 'The Return of the Protectorate': European elites co-opt their African counterparts in the 'co-management of flows', to prevent the latter's citizens from leaving. This would be an extension of projects already underway in Morocco and Libya, in which the elites themselves are granted free visas. And fifth, 'Bric-à-brac Politics': muddling through by means of a combination of small doses of all of the above, which is roughly speaking the status quo. Attempting to end on a slightly higher note, Smith appeals to the future of Africa: its youth are fleeing—or will be doing so in 2050—in order to liberate themselves, yet for the destiny of their continent they will be heading in the wrong direction: that energy would be better invested inward.

Smith's declared objective in *La ruée* is to provide 'a factual basis upon which each can raise up their own political tribune'. He pretends to a properly scientific stance: 'I am trying to evaluate the importance of Africa's reservoir of migrants and, as far as it is possible, to predict the scale of the flows that might be directed towards Europe, and their timing.' The sentence encapsulates a central weakness of Smith's book: his would-be sober objectivity rings hollow, because his very ontology—what he thinks he's looking at, the ways he carves up the social whole—already imbricate him in social and political webs that he never interrogates, and doesn't even acknowledge. Europeans seeing African people and land as a resource is not neutral: it has a long colonial history. Far from being a scholarly disquisition, *La ruée* is in fact a polemical squib, bearing all the hallmarks of the genre: hyperbole, scare tactics, selective use of facts. This is a rambling work, often frustratingly so. Smith has a tendency to raise a question, go off on a tangent and end with four paragraphs on an entirely different topic.

Dramatic exaggeration begins with the title. According to Smith, young Africa's mass migration north will represent 'an inversion' of the nineteenth-century 'scramble for Africa' by the European powers, when they apportioned the map of Africa at the 1885 Conference of Berlin. A scramble, then, is predatory: projecting African migrants as the protagonists of an imagined future rush to overpower the Europeans, demographically at least. It need hardly be said that the image is racialized, but Smith ladles it on. 'I do not lie awake at night trembling at the prospect of an "Africanization" of Europe', he insists, in the introduction to the English edition. But 'I can imagine how Europeans might quake at the thought'—and 'their fears are by no means groundless.'

According to demographic scholars and migration experts, 'groundless' is exactly what Smith's claims are. Although he thinks African demography 'has rarely aroused any curiosity or inspired any research'—his evidence for this comes from a Johns Hopkins post-grad reading list—his critics have pointed to the reams of existing work that Smith has overlooked. François Héran at INED, the French National Institute for Demographic Studies, signalled the glaring omission of the Global Bilateral Migration Database, a major source of knowledge on world diasporas. Michel Agier, an anthropologist at EHESS, the School of Advanced Studies in the Social Sciences, also questioned Smith's numbers. Seventy per cent of African migrants travel within the continent, and the preferred external destination is the US. Smith is just as selective with Sub-Saharan birth-rate figures. He fails to note that these have been on the decline since the mid-70s, already dropping from an average of 6.8 per woman then, to 4.8 in 2016 and trending down.

The parsimony of Smith's collective nouns—Europeans, Africans— elides and homogenizes the people they describe. His thesis is calibrated around the comparison of the two as demographic categories, but his generalizations and 'average figures' beg questions about the differences within them. The 15 per cent figure he cites for 'average' use of modern contraception masks wide variations within the continent—usage is over 60 per cent in South Africa, and generally much higher in the southern and eastern countries than in the West and Centre—and between city and rural dwellers. This is par for the course in Smith's selective treatment of facts. Examples are tossed in—high fertility levels in the hinterlands of northern Nigeria, for example—but whether they can be scaled up or accurately re-proportioned to represent Africa as a whole is never examined. Chastising Sub-Saharan rulers for their lack of 'demographic governance', he fails to engage with feminist critiques of technocratic attempts at fertility control, the history of colonial sterilization, male contraception or reproductive rights.

Crass tabloid tropes are dropped into the argument, by way of rhetorical flourish. Discussing the 'youth bulge' inspires Smith to lyrical flights about Africa as 'the island-continent of Peter Pan', 'a Neverland always in a state of becoming, without ever getting there'—'a "lost land" of failed adulthood, where hundreds of millions of castaways are waiting for a life of fulfilment beyond their reach.' His argument that youth represents a 'categorical inequality' that imperils Africa's democratic future ignores the frictive struggles to reclaim democratic forms all over the continent. He does not mention the youth movements in Senegal, Burkina Faso, South Africa, Congo, Angola and many other countries that are attempting to reclaim and rethink forms of participatory democracy. These young people do not imperil but rather seek to construct their countries' future. His Peter Pan rhetoric, figuring young people as impish and escapist, ignores the ways in which young Africans are political and social actors both within and beyond the boundaries of parliamentary politics. Democracy, in this book, appears to mean parliamentary liberal democracy, and Smith characterizes it as a pre-fabricated form that simply exists in the world—'there for the taking'. In truth, however, political forms cannot simply be applied in new places: they are renegotiated, adapted and contested. The idea of democracy as abstractly available is a technocratic fallacy, like his idea of 'good governance'.

Similarly, Africa remains conceptualized as a resource or repository for European ideas, rather than a site of theoretical, social and political innovation. Smith fails to engage with the ways in which histories of colonial capitalism have shaped international movements of labour. Meditating on why people migrate, Smith opines that young people want 'adventure', to 'catch a drop of luck', or to 'conquer or perish in universal time, in sync with the rest of the world'. There is no mention of the deleterious impact of Smith's lauded structural adjustment programmes—which drove large numbers of African professionals to the US and UK in the 1980s—nor of land-grabbing by agribusiness today. These occlusions are projected back in time. Africa's colonial past is given minimal significance: 'Colonialism only lasted about eighty years south of the Sahara. The "colonial imprint" cannot overwrite the longer history of the continent before and since.' Yet

Portugal, for example, dates its presence in Africa back to the 1400s. The Dutch arrived in Southern Africa in the seventeenth century; Mandela didn't come to power until 1994.

Rather than see Europe and Africa as connected in many ways, at different scales, through a unified but uneven economic system that European imperialism played a major role in establishing, he treats the two as entirely separate places connected through migration alone. To repurpose his lexicon, the problem is not that African young people are excluded from 'universal time', but rather that capitalist modernity manifests itself unevenly in different places. As Fredric Jameson remarked, we need to consider the Ford factory and the peasant field together. Smith's failure to address the economic system leads him to nebulous conclusions. He emphasizes that migration is only a possibility for people with some money (the very poorest cannot leave) and that the growing African middle classes will be better able to migrate. In the long term, Smith argues, it would be preferable for Africa to prosper, such that its population stays where it is. In the short term, however, Smith concludes that Europe is spending too much on development aid, which merely 'subsidizes migration'.

Smith is insistently communitarian, frequently emphasizing that it is up to Europe to decide who should be allowed across its borders. He doesn't address the inadequacy of this approach in dealing with the connected histories of Africa and Europe, or the economically extractive relations between them in the present. Europeans have not always subscribed to territorially bound conceptions of jurisdiction. It is not, as Smith puts it, 'irenic universalism' to take seriously the material and ethical implications of Europe's role in producing an unequal international system. Because he does not address the international division of labour, Smith depicts Africa as passive: it will 'continue to "be globalized" rather than take an active part in globalization'. He is silent on the dispersed histories of black and African labour in building European modernity. As Aimé Césaire wrote in Cahier d'un retour au pays natal: 'Bordeaux and Nantes and Liverpool and New York and San Francisco / Not an inch of this world devoid of my fingerprint.' If Smith could see African diasporas as productive rather than passive, it would be much more difficult for him to argue that migrants will dismantle European welfare states. Smith repeatedly presents migrants as 'guests' rather than as working, rights-bearing people, who contribute to and grow societies rather than deplete them.

In November 2018, Smith wrote a piece in Libération defending himself from claims that he was a lackey of the far right, after his work had been cited by anti-migrant polemics. But it is not the subject that makes his book open to such co-option so much as the way he develops his argument, carelessly deploying racialized stereotypes. Nigerians, we are told, resisted the colonial head tax with the same fervour as they did grasshopper swarms. Smith is not making the overtly racist analogy that Nigerians are like a swarm of insects, but, as with his concept of Africa's 'teeming youth', one can't but hear the double meanings in his text. Smith has a habit of making his arguments by deploying concepts, ideas and tropes that he apparently disagrees with. 'It is not necessarily *Lord of the Flies*, but . . .' 'The four-square native'—*le natif au carré*, 'a French person whose parents and grandparents were also French'—'has some excuse for thinking that France has long been a monochrome country.' Smith doesn't interrogate the implicit elision of legitimacy and race in the concept of the four-square native, though he says it's 'awkward'. If so, why insist on using it? The effect is a text in which these modes of thinking come to dominate. Despite Chirac's 'condescending infantilization' of Africa, he 'did make a valid point'. We may not share the former British Governor of Nigeria's motivations, but he did have 'great perspicacity'. Malthus has had a bad press, yet retains 'a bleak topicality'. I'm not a racist, but.

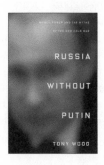

REVIEWS

Mauvaise Troupe Collective, *The ZAD and NoTAV: Territorial Struggles and the Making of a New Political Intelligence*
Translation and preface, Kristin Ross
Verso: London and New York 2018, $24.95, paperback
214 pp, 978 1 78663 496 2

REBECCA LOSSIN

MUTINOUS TERRITORY

The idea for a new French airport near Notre-Dame-des-Landes, a farming village some twelve miles northwest of Nantes, was originally floated in the late 1960s. Promoted by a regional bourgeoisie entranced by the modernization rhetoric of the post-war boom, it met immediate resistance from local farmers. Reasons for building the airport changed over the years—a touch-down point for Concorde, a third hub for the Greater Paris region, a real-estate bonanza for developers of Nantes' existing airport. Meanwhile, the re-classification of the six square-mile site as a *zone d'aménagement différé*, or ZAD, for eminent-domain purposes, allowed the state's solicitors to purchase land from farmers willing to sell and, in a sort of expropriation by attrition, to wait for other landowners to die. Put on hold during the economic crises of the late 1970s and 80s, the airport plan was resurrected in 2000 under Jospin. It was given official go-ahead in 2008, in the teeth of local opposition. That spring an old farmer, chatting to some local squatters during an anti-airport demonstration in Nantes, proposed that they come and occupy one of the empty farmsteads in the zone.

Over the next decade, a permanent encampment of activists flourished on the land, fighting off the development attempts by the French construction giant, Vinci. The occupiers recast the bureaucratic acronym ZAD as *la zad—zone à défendre*. At its height, the *zad* contained a bakery, a radio station, a newspaper, a bar, a website, spaces for musical performances, several subsistence farms and a market where no money changed hands. Yet the movement against the airport was decades in the making and the occupation only a late-stage crystallization in a process of multiple, intersecting forms of protest and organizing efforts that brought together farmers, squatters, anarchists, trade unionists, *nantais* citizens and elected local officials. It is more accurately described as a collective of organizations, ad hoc nature studies, investigative committees, farmworkers and other permanent residents, as well as members of the writing collective, Mauvaise Troupe.

In *ZAD and NoTAV*, the group pairs the experience of Notre-Dame-des-Landes with a parallel, ongoing struggle in Piedmont. The project for a high-speed train, or TAV—Italian: *treno ad alta velocità*—piercing the Alps between Lyon and Turin, was conceived by EU planners as part of Corridor Five, a mega-project for transport infrastructure that would arc from Lisbon to Kiev, to link the eastern and western flanks of the newly united continent. The TAV was scheduled to cut through the Val di Susa, running up from Turin to the French border—the route the Roman legions took into Gaul. Densely settled as it approaches Turin, studded with winter-sports resorts in its higher Alpine reaches, the Valley is a very different environment, geographically and socially, from the Loire-Atlantique—not least in its absorption through urban overspill of strains of Turin's traditional worker militancy. Yet the NoTAV campaign that sprang into being here in the 1990s confronted a nearly identical problem to the *zad*'s: the construction of redundant infrastructure.

Just as Nantes is home to a perfectly functional airport, an existing train line already operates, often at half-capacity, between Lyon and Turin. A giant motorway was constructed here in the 1980s, spanning the Valley on huge concrete struts, though it already possessed two national roads. In the words of Gianluca, a NoTAV pirate-radio operator, this is a territory 'midway between the mountains and the Turin periphery, even from the point of view of work—it must be the most industrialized, ruined, polluted, ravaged-by-infrastructure Alpine valley in all of Italy.' As with the *zad*, the NoTAV movement developed into an unlikely alliance between resistant villagers, ranging from pious Catholics to middle-aged ex-Maoists, and the young Turin *autonomia* and squatter milieus—a collaboration between dramatically contrasting political cultures. A signature of the movement has been its huge popular demonstrations, 80,000-strong, with village banners, tractors and icons of the Madonna of Rocciamelone making their way past rocks daubed 'TAV=Mafia', a reference to the big Italian construction interests involved.

ZAD and NoTAV is an elegant attempt to give a comparative account of these two sited struggles and to elicit the lessons in 'political intelligence' that they suggest. Mauvaise Troupe has already produced two shorter books on the *zad* and an earlier compilation of stories and pictures from other alter-globo and anti-austerity struggle sites, mainly in France. Based on over a hundred interviews conducted in the Val Di Susa and Notre-Dame-des-Landes in 2014–15, *ZAD and NoTAV* is an attractively written hybrid of amateur ethnography and reportage, buttressed by first-person accounts, opening out into a set of speculations on 'the people' and 'the popular', the relations between the different components of these 'communities in struggle', the uses and abuses of the territories involved, and the potential diffusion of such forms of resistance. It's nicely translated here by Kristin Ross, American scholar of French history and literature, author of landmark works on Rimbaud, May 68 and the Paris Commune, and a supporter of the *zad* since she was invited there for a discussion on communal luxury. Her informative introduction sets the *zad* and NoTAV in the context of protest occupations from Japan's Narita Airport and the Xingu River dam in Brazil to the Standing Rock Sioux's resistance to the North Dakota Pipeline.

One of the many signs erected on the *zad* reads, 'Against the Airport and its World'. With the establishment of a successful communal living arrangement, the possibility of an alternative took on a concrete form and the airport assumed a metonymic function in the thought-world of the occupiers. The attempt to register such an alternative makes for an odd book, resistant to summary. The opening section, criss-crossing between Brittany and Piedmont, provides an over-arching double narrative of the two. It is not easy, however, to disentangle the territory from the people, or the forms of protest—barricades, sabotage—from the logistics of occupation and defence, and these also resist division at the textual level. The book's structure reflects the attempt to negotiate the untranslatable reality of a territory where the meaning of nature itself was undergoing many simultaneous transformations. The land chosen for the airport had been referred to as both a swamp and a desert by developers. As a result of political struggle, it was discovered that it was in fact a biodiverse wetland.

The proper designation of this muddy landscape is *bocage*, a borrowed word meaning 'little woods', the product of feudal property arrangements. Flat farming land, it is broken up by hedges, shrubs and clusters of trees that record a human footprint made by a pre-capitalist peasantry. It also memorializes the end of communal land usage in Brittany, for the hedgerows were instruments of enclosure. *Bocage* as an environmental designation thus contains a politically relevant history of land use—and it is land use, in several senses, that is documented and conceptualized in this text. The re-zoning of the area changed the landscape yet again. It is because much of it was taken out of use as farmland in the 1970s that the ZAD became such a rich site of biodiversity, while the surrounding areas fell prey to agricultural modernization. The construction company and its boosters in the regional government responded with a green-washing campaign. They promised an airport that would aim at 'optimal integration with the landscape'. Single-storied and covered with a 'vegetalized' roof, 'the terminal will appear like a section of the bocage that rises up'.

To the authors' delight, the *bocage*, in all its historical and natural density, did rise up. The Loire-Atlantique region was a stronghold of the French worker-farmers movement, Paysans travailleurs, that arose amid the broader upheavals of 1968, memorably theorized by local sharecropper Bernard Lambert, in *Les Paysans dans la lutte des classes* (1970). Lambert was one of the leaders of the farmers' march to occupy the Larzac plateau and celebrated its 'marriage' with the ongoing occupation of the Lip watch factory as an alliance of rural and urban proletariats. The Confederation Paysanne, a radical union of agricultural workers that emerged from this tradition in the late 1980s, would provide crucial support to the struggle against the airport when the project was resuscitated in 2000. It was joined by a local citizens' association, ACIPA, and an umbrella organization known as the Coordination that brought together over fifty groups opposed to the project.

From the beginning, the campaign exceeded a stereotypically rural conservatism. Like most infrastructure projects, the airport at Notre-Dame-des-Landes had been sold as a great economic boon to local inhabitants. Early activism positioned itself against the economized world of the airport rather than in defence of tradition and, to that end, began a series of counter-investigations to show that the airport would do more than eliminate farms. Local shopkeepers and café owners hoped to profit from increased traffic to the region, so activists travelled to Roissy to record the noise levels at Charles de Gaulle Airport and interview people who lived and worked in its vicinity: 'We were able to show that the corner café had closed because passengers went to the airport café and the village was dead.'

In the Val di Susa, too, resistance began with environmental-impact studies. These were conducted by a local group called Habitat, which could draw on expertise from the University of Turin and had already organized against an arms factory sited in its village. Habitat likewise recorded the noise of high-speed trains and investigated the problems with asbestos in the mountain-sides through which the TAV construction engineers would be drilling. It produced a mass of popular educational material to take round the villages. The Valley's previous experiences with large-scale infrastructure projects also underwrote its definitive 'no' to the TAV. In the 1980s, villagers had been taken in by false promises that the motorway would be 'ecological' and provide local jobs, which failed to materialize. A few years later, they organized successfully against the construction of a 400,000-volt overhead power-line that would have connected the Valley to the Superphénix nuclear reactor in France. The Valsusians had refused to allow local politicians to take over the leadership of that campaign. 'We delegated nothing', a 69-year-old villager recalled. 'They were free to come with us, but we had direct control. It was the right way to go about things and in the end we won.'

Villagers cited the power-line victory as the model for NoTAV, whose basic unit has been the village-level *comitato di lotta popolare*. The terminology of popular struggle reflects the militant recent past in the region: a dozen members of Prima Linea were arrested there in the 1970s. But Mauvaise Troupe emphasizes intimate and immediate concerns as the main point of departure for the radical NoTAV movement. Stefano, a 57-year-old member of the Bussaleno popular struggle committee, put it this way:

> I was a political militant, I spent eight years in prison. But I'm from here, I love nature—ecologist is not the right word but yes, I'm connected with nature. The TAV bothers me personally . . . It's not because it represents capital and I'm a communist I'm against it. No. It's because it devastates the valley for me, it surrounds me with asbestos, it's disgusting, and I'm fighting it for those reasons.

But intimacy, immediacy and personal interest should not be confused with a necessarily apolitical position. One of the virtues of this testimony is its demonstration of the porousness of the personal and the political. The accounts of the participants makes it clear that 'those reasons' frequently gave way to broader ideological investments. Likewise, quotidian forms of activism such as committee membership and peaceful protest were often transformed through confrontations with police violence or by increased first-hand knowledge into a militant opposition. It would be wildly inaccurate to describe the account of these movements conveyed in *ZAD and NoTAV* as 'not ideological', but the coupling of first-hand accounts with explanatory text does effectively demonstrate a politics in process constituted by individual participants, rather than a political programme formulated in advance. It models many different ways into a robust, participatory politics.

Jasmin's account is a good illustration. She arrived at the *zad* as 'more of a naturalist than a militant', with the intention of making an inventory of wildlife and a map of the area. As media attention increased, more naturalists arrived to study the flora and fauna of the *bocage*. Eventually they formed a group, Naturalists in Struggle. Like many components of the *zad* and the larger anti-airport campaign, it was at once a satellite of long-standing naturalist organizations in the region and something new—qualitatively altered by the context of the battle. As Jasmin put it, this was 'the first time that we were exercising our passion in the framework of a struggle'. She ended up living on the *zad* for two years, during which time she led botanical tours. The *zad* didn't simply supply an invigorating framework for the naturalists' endeavours. Their inventories identified rare species that were dependent on its unique habitat. This allowed for legal claims, as well as a more developed critique of the airport company's green-washing. Mauvaise Troupe notes the 'glaring contradiction' of the Hollande government's promotion of a new airport while at the same time 'bragging about hosting the world-wide climate summit'. The naturalists took issue with the very idea of 'environmental compensation' and, with record-keeping that would appear apolitical in any other context, provided a detailed material argument against 'the conversion of biodiversity into a monetary value'.

Years of diligent legal protests and alternative studies organized by Coordination and ACIPA having failed to block the onset of construction works, resistance took a more militant turn. With the call by tenant farmers, local protesters—*les habitant.e.s qui resistent*—and squatters for a full-scale occupation, the non-negotiable 'no' of the anti-airport activists was given a concrete form. In the summer of 2009, radical anti-capitalist ecologists and degrowth militants organized a Climate Action Camp in the *zad*, while the *habitant.e.s* called for more occupiers to come and build dwellings there. In 2011, *zadistes* toured urban squatting scenes, calling for more support. The historic presence of the worker-farmer movement was highly visible in the tractors that now functioned as movable barricades against the police and construction crews. Access roads were constantly guarded.

There were continuous skirmishes between occupiers and the company's subcontractors. Militants targeted the equipment of Biotope, the 'green-washing mercenaries' hired by the developers. Shoyu, a member of a vegan cookery collective, describes how the masked occupiers repeatedly sabotaged Biotope's collection of soil samples, stole their paperwork and slashed their vehicles' tyres. The regional media attacked the 'riff-raff' living on the site, with some backing from Green Party members. Trials of some of the activists began in Nantes, countered by a 10,000-strong anti-airport demonstration, flanked by 200 tractors. The territory itself was re-shaped by defensive considerations. As *ZAD and NoTAV* explains, the first dwellings built on the *zad* were 'strewn across the zone without any logical coherence, making a collective defence difficult to imagine'. The occupiers now began to think strategically about the space as they considered how best to prepare for the police—mapping the area, testing communications systems. Characteristically, this had a whimsical aspect. One occupier describes the planning of a garden in terms of resisting eviction: 'We put barbed wire across the rear entry points, we tried to lay out the plantings so that the first things to be destroyed would not be the tomatoes.'

In October 2012 the Préfecture launched Operation Caesar, aiming to raze the *zad* with the help of bulldozers and 1,200 riot police. Outside supporters rushed to the site; farmers opened their homes. *ZAD and NoTAV* gives a vivid account of the epic battles during those weeks: farmers threw up barricades of telegraph poles and hay bales to halt the police advance as temporary dwellings and vegetable gardens were bulldozed and heavy armoured vehicles sank in the mud. New dwellings were hastily built, the copse 'ringing with the sound of hammers'. Police occupied the cross-roads at the main entrance to the site all through the winter. When they finally withdrew in the spring of 2014, there was an explosion of activity on the *zad*—a new influx of occupiers, plantings, mass events. When the developers tried to start exploratory drilling work again the following year, a demonstration of 60,000, including five hundred tractors, took over the centre of Nantes. Construction of the airport was indefinitely postponed, pending legal appeals, although there would be further attempts at eviction.

In Val di Susa, exploratory vertical drilling for the TAV tunnel began in the late 1990s, despite the local protests. Soon after, nocturnal sabotage attacks commenced against the company's equipment, accompanied by 'obscure' graffiti—an odd mix of anti-capitalism and racism—that to the vil-lagers suggested provocateurs. A little later, three anarchists were arrested in a Turin squat, accused of the attacks and charged with 'terrorist aims'. Held in solitary confinement, one was found dead in his cell; another killed her-self a few months later. Mauvaise Troupe argues that the alliances between Turin's radical youth milieu and the NoTAV movement intensified after their deaths: 'the valley demonstrated in the city', and summer camps in the mountains introduced the city's young to the valley's struggle. In 2003, the company began setting up sites to extract soil samples, endowing the project with a visible reality. But legibility is double-edged and opponents now had a target. Tens of thousands marched against the drilling sites, broke in and occupied them. In 2005, the protesters occupying a new site in a field above the valley established a permanent encampment—a *presidio*, or garrison. Patrizia, a 57-year-old cook: 'The first morning we just had a few seats and a picnic table. The next day we had an umbrella and two tents'—and 'little by little', a wooden mountain hut.

That October, protesters confronted riot police on a bridge over a water-fall, high up the mountain. Nicoletta, a 69-year-old member of the Bussoleno popular struggle committee:

> There were just a hundred of us—we were sandwiched. The police had taken down the railings of the bridge and the waterfall was a few metres below us. They could have killed us. But a miracle happened and we began to see lights arriving from all sides of the mountain. The hundred of us stood our ground, and then . . . the whole mountain came alive, with people coming to join us. In an instant there were a thousand of us and things looked a bit different!

The stand-off at Seghino Bridge was followed by a valley-wide insurrection in December 2005, when word went round that construction work was start-ing at Venaus, high up by the French border. Riot police demolished the NoTAV *presidio* in the middle of a snowy night, clubbing the fifty occupiers.

By dawn, there were church bells ringing, firemen sounding their sirens, municipal police using their cars' loudspeakers to rally against the *carabinieri*. Mauvaise Troupe detail the spontaneous general strike that brought schoolchildren as much as shopkeepers out into the streets, protesters throwing up barricades across the motorway, the 70,000-strong march that chased the *carabinieri* from the construction site. With the 2006 Turin Winter Olympics fast approaching, the Berlusconi government called a temporary halt to TAV construction that would last for the next four years.

Collectively authored, unsure of its tense, at once polemical and documentary, *ZAD and NoTAV* is an odd book, but in its own way compelling for just that reason. As an attempt to write a comparative, subjectively informed account of two ongoing movements through the incorporation of a number of genres, it enacts a sort of methodological challenge appropriate to its topic. As a result, its reflective double chronicle has not been dated by subsequent events. In January 2018 the Macron government announced that the new airport would not be built at Notre-Dame-des-Landes, though former *zadistes* continue to negotiate with the French authorities over the use of the land. The NoTAV campaign has yet to win anything so definitive from the Italian state. In opposition, the Five Stars Movement gave NoTAV its full backing and won the support of many voters in the region. In office it has so far blocked the tendering process on the Italian side, amid calls for a referendum on the TAV. Since 2011, however, the European Commission has thrown its full weight behind the project—a point missed by Mauvaise Troupe—and 40 per cent of the Lyon–Turin link will be funded by the EU. On the French side of the border there has been no corresponding NoTAV movement and work there has proceeded on schedule.

What insights does Mauvaise Troupe glean from all this for 'the making of a new political intelligence'? *ZAD and NoTAV* offers no portable political programme, no directions for running communal farms, although it suggests a number of exemplary transpositions: *zad* for ZAD, political affinities for power-lines, barricades for farming equipment, precious territory for useless swamp, solidarity for NIMBYism. At the core of this demonstrative rather than programmatic strategy is the alternative internationalism posited by the connection between the *zad* and the NoTAV movements. In both instances, the defence of a territory altered existing forms of sociality and in some cases produced entirely new ones. Nicoletta, the protester on the Seghino Bridge, summarizes the experience in Val di Susa: 'There were oldsters, people from the popular struggle committee, but there were also many young people who had started to come from elsewhere, because they found here a way to satisfy the need for opposition that they couldn't find anywhere else.'

Yet one strength of Mauvaise Troupe's approach is the careful attention the collective pays to the distinctions between the two campaigns. In Val di Susa, concepts of 'the popular' and 'the people' were self-explanatory. At Notre-Dame-des-Landes, they were distrusted. The idea of a republican people that emerged from the French Revolution was quickly neutralized by the installation of the bourgeoisie, ZAD and NoTAV argues, and later 'worked over, stabilized and integrated into a vast system of democratic governance'. A homogenizing fiction, it allowed no internal contradiction, ethical divergence or differential relationship to power. Yet the act of governing also included the capacity to designate and excommunicate 'internal enemies' remobilizing the abstraction of a united people against them. In late 2015, the conjunction of terrorist attacks in Paris and a fresh police assault on the zad threw these tensions into relief. As Hollande imposed a state of emergency, the media and political establishment exhorted the 'French people' to identify with the 'Bataclan generation'—'open, hedonistic, flexible'—against 'the terrorists', an enemy that could easily extend to any migrant and all Muslims. No other division could be allowed. As Mauvaise Troupe has it, the zadistes and their allies defied Hollande's ban on demonstrations to set out on tractors and bicycles to protest in the spirit of the Communards against the heads of government gathered for the Paris climate summit at Versailles.

ZAD and NoTAV acknowledges the contradictions inherent in the zad's attempts at prefigurative politics: 'The defeat of a police operation will never be enough to destroy what remains of the grip of consumerism within us, the devastating addictions, the prejudices, the everyday sexism.' And yet, actually existing commoning was a reality for almost ten years. The political challenge of living communally, commented upon and recorded throughout the book, is summarized at one point as the 'problem of the one and the multiple'. It is a problem that the authors have no interest in definitively resolving. This generative instability is spatially encoded as well. While there were monthly General Assembly meetings at the Vacherit, there was no designated space for decision-making on the zad. The 'composition' of the different 'components' into a 'community of struggle' was not easy to sustain, outside moments of high tension. Often the result was 'conjugated actions', with each group promoting its own chosen tactic: counter-expertise, direct action, non-violence, hunger strike, sabotage. The authors assert that neither a 'democratic imaginary' nor 'the search for a consensus as an ideal' were suited to the political tasks of living on the zad. 'Real finesse' was required if aspirations were to reinforce rather than neutralize each other. There were sharp differences over both sabotage and street violence as tactics, with local inhabitants complaining the occupiers were inviting police repression. Yet attitudes shifted when it came to building barricades against police invasion.

Communal sociality looks different in the Val di Susa, but living in protest is living differently. If there is no autonomous 'lawless zone', the landscape still changes for people involved in NoTAV. One member explains the strange appearance of a tourist bus at a TAV construction site: 'They are Valsusians returning from a seaside outing, but before going back to their homes they come by to scream their rage.' Here the negotiations between different political cultures involved greater recognition of the other's point of view. Luca, a young militant, speaks of the importance for the Valsusians of 'the legitimacy of numbers'. Anarchists would undertake an action with five people, or two. Valsusians 'are used to being very numerous—thirty or forty thousand for the marches, so if there's a hundred, they'll say, "Something isn't right, where are all the others? If they aren't here, it means they don't agree."' The idea of legitimacy was hard to define—'it's a combination of a sense of justice, the emotion in the moment, and the number of people'— but 'it's what guides many of the practices of the Valsusian struggle.'

Sylvia Federici has argued that primitive accumulation should be understood not simply as an early stage of capitalism, but an on-going process. New enclosures have made communal property and relations that were assumed extinct visible once again. Ross suggests that recent examples of robust political organizing are tied to the land through their recognition of the catastrophic climate change that will, as a result of enclosure, make living together on Earth into an impossibility. This makes the commons once again visible and more necessary. *ZAD and NoTAV* is a notable book for this reason. It demonstrates that the defence of a literal, sited commons is at once a refusal of the wealth transfer entailed in state-sponsored land-grabs and a necessary component of maintaining political alternatives by exerting control over the means of social reproduction. A record of lived experience rather than an abstract manifesto, it carries a corresponding degree of conviction. In spite of the absence of an articulated programme, it is also a galvanizing text in its demonstration of the entanglement of militant actions and the reproduction of everyday life. And the presence of multiple, visible voices, rather than the all-knowing anonymity of competing political tracts like the Invisible Committee's *The Coming Insurrection*, is both politically and formally important.

There are, of course, unavoidable questions of representation and the first-person narratives cannot completely displace the suspicion that at least a few things are being misrepresented here. Mauvaise Troupe undertakes no critical reflection on its own 'components' and their 'composition'. We are told only that the collective has 'varied in number'. Nor is there any attempt to provide a more detailed analysis of the class characters of the regions and the economic relations involved. It is difficult, for example, not to see a conflict between the large and petty bourgeoisie as a much more significant factor in the protest against the airport, and one wonders what impact the presence of occupiers could have on the political consciousness of small-business owners. At the same time, the book is full of astonishing stories, vignettes that may be testaments to the efficacy of commoning as a means of political transformation—a man emerging from a BMW, pulling a chainsaw out of its trunk and asking which tree he should cut down for the barricade, for example. Or a farmer, after working on the *zad*, suddenly finding it bizarre to hear a friend demand that his wife make drinks for them.

The history of militant action in Italy, and broader reactions to it, is also insufficient. It is not a coincidence that the NoTAV struggle is happening near Turin. It would also be useful to know more about the regional political situation in the Loire-Atlantique and the actions taken by ACIPA and the other groups that were waging a war of attrition long before the *zad* was founded. The question of how one maintains a communal life in struggle beyond the moment of conflict or maintains a commune in acute opposition to authorities—in a state of permanent defence—without eventually succumbing to authoritarian tendencies is crucial and an attention to these other, less radical but also less romantic forms of struggle, could be helpful here. But to paraphrase Marx on the Paris Commune, the most significant thing about the *zad* is that it happened, and a record of this happening is good to have.